Blueprint for Use of Nursing Models

Blueprint for Use of Nursing Models

Education, Research, Practice, and Administration

Patricia Hinton Walker
Betty Neuman

Editors

NLN Press • New York
Pub. No. 14-2696

The views expressed in this book reflect those of the authors and do not necessarily reflect the official views of the National League for Nursing.

Library of Congress Cataloging-in-Publication Data

Blueprint for use of nursing models / Patricia Hinton Walker, Betty Neuman, editors.
       p.   cm. — (Pub. : no. 14-2696)
    Includes bibliographical references.
    ISBN 0-88737-656-8
    1. Nursing models.   I. Walker, Patricia Hinton.   II. Neuman, Betty M.   III. Series: Pub. (National League for Nursing) : no. 14-2696.
    [DNLM: 1. Models, Nursing.   WY 20.5 B658 1996]
RT84.5.B58   1996
610.73'01'1—dc20
DNLM/DLC
for Library of Congress   96-19656
                                                               CIP

This book was set in Garamond by Publications Development Company, Crockett, Texas. The designer was Allan Graubard. The printer was Book Crafters. The cover was designed by Lauren Stevens.

Printed in the United States of America.

Contents

Contributors   *vii*

Preface   *xi*

Foreword   *xv*

SECTION I THE BLUEPRINT

1   **Blueprint for Selection and Implementation
    of Nursing Models**   **3**
    Patricia Hinton Walker and Betty Neuman

2   **Blueprint Example: An Integrated Model for
    Evaluation, Research, and Policy Analysis in the
    Context of Managed Care**   **11**
    Patricia Hinton Walker

SECTION II BLUEPRINTS FOR RESEARCH

3   **The Johnson Behavioral System Model:
    Explaining Activities of Chronically Ill Children**   **33**
    *Bonnie Holaday, Anne Turner-Henson,
    and James Swan*

4   **The Roy Adaptation Model in Research:
    Rehabilitation Nursing**   **64**
    Stacey Hoffman Barone and Callista Roy

SECTION III BLUEPRINTS FOR EDUCATION

5   **The Neuman Systems Model in
    Nursing Education**   **91**
    *Victoria Strickland Seng, Rosalie Mirenda,
    and Lois W. Lowry*

6   Watson's Theory of Transpersonal Caring   141
    M. Jean Watson

SECTION IV   BLUEPRINTS FOR PRACTICE

7   Levine's Conservation Model: Caring for
    Women with Chronic Illness   187
    Karen Moore Schaefer

8   Application of Self-Care Deficit
    Nursing Theory   228
    *Ruben D. Fernandez, George J. Hebert,
    and Jane Bliss-Holtz*

9   The Riehl Interaction Model   236
    Joan Riehl

SECTION V   BLUEPRINTS FOR ADMINISTRATION

10 Nursing Administration and the Neuman
    Systems Model   251
    Dorothy Craig and Charlene Beynon

11 Computerization of Self-Care Deficit Nursing
    Theory in a Medical Center   275
    Jane Bliss-Holtz and Joanne Riggs

SECTION VI   INTERNATIONAL BLUEPRINT
             APPLICATION

12 The Roper–Logan–Tierney Model: A Model in
    Nursing Practice   289
    *Nancy Roper, Winifred Logan,
    and Alison Tierney*

SECTION VII   THE FUTURE

13 Theory Development: A Blueprint for the
    21st Century   317
    Afaf I. Meleis

Index   *331*

Contributors

**Stacey Hoffman Barone,
PhD, RN, CRRN**
Clinical Nurse Researcher
New England Rehabilitation
    Hospital
Woburn, MA

Charlene Beynon, MscN
Assistant Director of Nursing
Education & Research Division
Middlesex-London Health Unit
London, Ontario
Canada
Assistant Professor
University of Western Ontario
London, Ontario
Canada

Jane Bliss-Holtz, DNSc, RN
Assistant Director of Nursing
Newark Beth Israel Medical
    Center
Newark, NJ
Assistant Professor
Rutgers, the State University of
    New Jersey
College of Nursing
Newark, NJ

Dorothy Craig, MScN, RN
Professor
Faculty of Nursing
University of Toronto
Toronto, Ontario
Canada

**Ruben D. Fernandez, PhD
Candidate, MA, BSN**
Vice President–Nursing
Newark Beth Israel Medical
    Center
Newark, NJ

George J. Hebert, MA, BSN, RN
Assistant Director
Christ Hospital
School of Nursing
Jersey City, NJ

**Bonnie Holaday, DNS, RN,
FAAN**
Professor & Chair
School of Nursing
Wichita State University
Wichita, KS

**Winifred Logan, MA, DNS
(Educ), RGN, RNT**
East Grange
St. Andrews
Scotland, UK

Lois W. Lowry, DNSc, RN
Associate Professor
University of South Florida
College of Nursing
Health Sciences Center
Tampa, FL

**Afaf Ibrahim Meleis, RN,
PhD, DrPs (Hon)**
Professor
School of Nursing
Department of Mental Health,
  Community and Administrative
  Nursing
University of California
San Francisco, CA

Rosalie Mirenda, DNSc, RN
Vice President for Academic
  Affairs and Professor, Nursing
Neumann College
Aston, PA

Betty Neuman, PhD, FAAN
Theorist–Consultant
Founder/Director, Neuman
  Systems Model
Beverly, OH

Joan Riehl, PhD, RN
Author, Lecturer, Consultant
Riehl Interaction Model
Los Angeles, CA

Joanne Riggs, RN, MA
Director of Nursing
Newark Beth Israel Medical Center
Newark, NJ

**Nancy Roper, MPhil, SRN,
RSCN, RNT**
Author, Lecturer
Edinburgh
Scotland, UK

**Sr. Callista Roy, PhD, RN,
FAAN**
Professor & Nurse Theorist
Boston College
Chestnut Hill, MA

**Karen Moore Schaefer, RN,
DNSc**
Associate Professor
Allentown College of St. Francis de
  Sales
Center Valley, PA

**Victoria Strickland Seng,
PhD, RN**
Chair & Associate Professor
University of Tennessee at Martin
Department of Nursing
Martin, TN

James H. Swan, PhD
Associate Professor
Department of Health Services
  Organization & Policy
Wichita State University
Wichita, KS

Alison Tierney, BSc(SocSc-Nurs), PhD, RGN
Department of Nursing
  Studies
Adam Ferguson Building
University of Edinburgh
George Square
Edinburgh
Scotland, UK

Anne Turner-Henson, DSN, RN
Associate Professor
School of Nursing
University of Alabama
Birmingham, AL

Patricia Hinton Walker, PhD, FAAN
Associate Professor
University of Rochester and
Kate Hanna Harvey, Visiting
  Professor
Frances Payne Bolton
School of Nursing
Case Western Reserve University
Cleveland, OH

M. Jean Watson, PhD, RN, FAAN
Distinguished Professor of Nursing
Director–Center for Human Caring
University of Colorado
School of Nursing
Denver, CO

Preface

*T*his book provides linkages to nursing's rich past, is relevant to the present, and offers guidance for future use of nursing models into the 21st century. Because it is a comprehensive book featuring practical applications of nursing theorists' work, this blueprint serves as a needed resource to students, clinical practitioners, nursing faculty, researchers, and administrators. The book's value in a global health market is enhanced by its international contributions. The generic nature of the book will inform and invite cooperation and inquiry from other disciplines, and will educate them about the value of nursing's holistic approach to health. In the future, expanded views and theoretical structures will be needed to facilitate new knowledge development and to address a changing world's health concerns, outcomes, roles, and relationships. The editors anticipate that this book will act as a springboard for a new generation of innovative thinkers and scholars who will explore interdisciplinary, philosophical, and creative conceptualizations.

A unique feature of this book is that leading nursing theorists either chose to write their chapters or delegated the writing to a model-user of their choice. Whether written or sanctioned by the theorists, these chapters faithfully reflect their views. The theorists' support is evident in an introductory paragraph at the beginning of each delegated chapter. The editors invited all major theorists to participate in this book, but conflicts prohibited some contributions in the time allotted, and a few invited authors elected not to participate for various other reasons. Chapters describing theorists' work are organized within each section in alphabetical order. In a few cases, the decision to include relevant topics such as informatics, community health, and health policy created the need to focus on the work of a particular theorist in more than one chapter. Some theorists' work is presented more comprehensively and reflects broader use, beyond education, practice, research, or administration. For readers' benefit, examples of where and how the theorists' models are being used are listed at the end of each chapter. The final chapter highlights future implications for nursing model implementation within the changing health care arena.

The book is intended to provide a blueprint for the use of nursing models—a guide that will assist individuals and organizations to utilize nursing models within a variety of settings. Sections of the book are designed for functional use by readers seeking to implement nursing models in research, education, practice, and administration worldwide. The editors purposefully limited each section to two or three contributions in order to simplify the process of learning to implement a model within the above chosen area. The first chapter in Section I, **The Blueprint,** is designed to assist readers in determining the fit of a particular model and suggests plans for successful implementation of a nursing model in selected settings, projects, and/or populations. The example in the second chapter serves two purposes: (a) explicating the value and use of the blueprint for a nursing model and (b) demonstrating how the blueprint can assist scholars to expand a nursing model into futuristic integrative models. The chapter also highlights model use in relation to costing, health risk, care across the continuum, and health policy. Meleis, in the final chapter, identifies these factors as essential to model use in the future.

Two outstanding examples of implementation of nursing models for research are featured in Section II, **Blueprints for Research.** These chapters offer excellent demonstrations of how nursing models can be effectively used in clinical research. Chapter 3 highlights solid clinical research methodology and focuses on care of chronically ill children, using Johnson's Behavioral System Model. Chapter 4, coauthored by Stacey Hoffman Barone and theorist Callista Roy, provides an excellent discussion of the use of both qualitative and quantitative research designs and presents research related to rehabilitation nursing.

Section III, **Blueprints for Education,** describes implementations of nursing models, from basic to advanced levels, in a variety of institutions. Chapter 5 presents implementation strategies for both baccalaureate and associate degree settings, using the Neuman Systems Model. Chapter 6 is a comprehensive treatment of the Theory of Transpersonal Caring. Author–theorist Jean M. Watson focuses primarily on education and describes common uses of the caring paradigm for both entry and advanced levels of learning. Watson presents applications of her model in a practice setting and has included important literature references.

Section IV, **Blueprints for Practice,** presents three applications of nursing models in practice settings. Chapter 7, a comprehensive chapter on the care of chronically ill women, describes Levine's Conservation Model. A detailed plan of implementation of Orem's Self-Care Deficit Nursing Theory in an acute care practice setting is presented in Chapter 8. Several case examples of how the care of women and children was effected using the Riehl Interaction Model are described in Chapter 9, authored by theorist Joan Riehl.

For Section V, **Blueprints for Administration,** two chapters were selected to address emerging areas in health care. The content of these chapters differs significantly, yet each clearly demonstrates the relevance of administrators' use of nursing models in community health and nursing informatics. Chapter 10, a Canadian contribution, describes implementation of the Neuman Systems Model at both a regional public health division and a district mental health center. The coauthors' attention to detail from an administrator's perspective is commendable. Chapter 11, the other entry in this section, addresses a critical need for nursing. Orem's Self-Care Deficit Nursing Theory is used as a framework for development and implementation of a nursing information system designed to support clinical practice.

Sections VI and VII, titled **International Blueprint Application** and **The Future,** respectively, enhance the book's content by expanding traditional approaches and thinking related to the use of nursing models. In Chapter 12, Roper, Logan, and Tierney present their Activities for Living Model, a nursing model developed in England and used in Europe. The chapter introduces a global perspective of nursing and describes components relevant to health care worldwide: the dependence/independence continuum and the lifespan. The model has been implemented in a large practice setting that includes groups of hospitals and services. A thoughtful concluding chapter by Afaf Meleis encourages expanding the nursing profession to explore theory development and the use of nursing models in the future. Meleis clearly articulates the value of the nursing model, but challenges future models' users and developers to expand their thinking and model structures into the 21st century.

PATRICIA HINTON WALKER AND BETTY NEUMAN

Foreword

A blueprint gives us direction; it provides an outline, detailing the structure and boundaries of a system. The authors of this *Blueprint* aim to provide direction for the discipline of nursing, to guide the development of scientific thinking in nursing education, practice, research, and administration. Included are a range of topics, each from a nursing conceptualization, but each with specific details and examples of applications. This text goes a step beyond what has been available in the literature. By adding depth to the nursing perspective, it will guide future graduate students to make the necessary connections between nursing conceptual models and their own day-to-day experiences of nursing, whether at a patient's bedside or at a computer terminal where they are designing the clinical information system for a target project.

In the initial chapter, Patricia Hinton Walker and Betty Neuman explicate the guidelines for model selection and implementation. They raise critical issues that are addressed in subsequent chapters: the fit of the conceptual model to the setting; the purpose of the model, and the relationship of this purpose to the planned use of the model; and the relationship of the model to the political, cultural, and social setting. A concept analysis framework is proposed to assist in further defining the model's key features in relation to the setting and/or organization. The authors then pose a series of important questions that help to frame the subsequent analyses—questions that are closely oriented to the structure of the models. This internal analysis is followed by a model for external analysis, that is, the application of the model to specific practice, research, or administration situations. Two additional structured models extend the analysis to organizational development and strategic planning. Chapter 2 presents an example of a blueprint: an integrated model and its relevance in the context of managed care.

This key section, which sets the format, guidelines, and tone for the book, is followed by five application sections covering, respectively: research, education, practice, administration, and international. Examples are drawn from a selection of nursing conceptual models. The concluding section projects the challenging disciplinary issues for the 21st century, recognizing, at the same time, the progress made thus far in delineating nursing science.

This book will be welcomed especially by graduate students and practicing nurses who are seeking expansion of their understanding of the conceptualizations that form the basis for professional nursing behavior. Other disciplines may benefit as well. Important questions are raised by the contributors, questions that will stimulate further inquiry and discovery and will ultimately enhance better nursing and health care interventions.

JOYCE J. FITZPATRICK, PhD, FAAN

Section I

The Blueprint

Blueprint for Selection and Implementation of Nursing Models

Patricia Hinton Walker and Betty Neuman

*T*his blueprint for selection and implementation of nursing models, given below in outline form, is designed to be used as a guide for students, practitioners, administrators, educators, and researchers who are interested in implementing nursing theoretical models within a variety of settings. In preparing the blueprint, we have taken a position consistent with Meleis (1995): "[N]ursing conceptualizations are theories that can be used to describe and prescribe different aspects of nursing care. They are not competing models; they are complementing theories that may provide a conceptualization of different aspects, components, or concepts of the domain" (p. 17).

Consequently, this blueprint will provoke important questions that should be asked about the fit of a particular model to a person, purpose, and setting.

An architectural blueprint of a projected structure allows a builder or prospective owner to view simultaneously all areas of the architect's design. A wise builder or investor will review the foundation area first, to be certain that it is firmly placed and anchored, contains correct materials and design, and will offer the necessary support to the other areas of the structure with predictable outcomes. With a solid foundation ensured, the other areas of the structure can be reviewed in the sequence given by the architect or in a sequence that is of more immediate interest. Our blueprint can be viewed in the same way. Area I is comparable to a structure's foundation: answers to the questions in this Area will determine whether the other Areas can be reasonably considered. We encourage moving through the Areas of our blueprint in the sequence we have established, but, knowing how diverse the applications of our blueprint can be, we acknowledge that Areas II through VI may be validated in a different sequence or may have varying levels of precedence. We advise reading the entire blueprint before deciding whether its sequence, in Areas II through VI, would be more applicable in a revised order.

Areas I and II encourage readers to investigate philosophical underpinnings and explore the concepts/subconcepts of the particular model of choice. This can be done by conducting an in-depth review of a theorist's work—that is, by searching the literature for specific examples of implementation of the particular model of interest. We also recommend that potential users of nursing models review one of the many texts that provide a conceptual analysis of the leading models. Authors of sources about conceptual approaches and nursing theory include: Fawcett (1989), Leddy and Pepper, (1993), Meleis (1991), and Oermann (1991).

Area III addresses the more practical questions to be considered before attempting to implement a model. Many theorists (and the book's editors) have received numerous telephone calls, questions, and requests for consultation on use of nursing models. Because potential users often seek very specific information about how to implement models, we offer here a listing of practical questions to be considered before attempting to implement a model. From experience, we know that a well-thought-out plan considers education, development of tools, and potential costs for implementing a nursing model with groups in practice, education, administration, and/or research.

Areas IV and V specifically address needs of potential model users who plan to implement a nursing model on an organizational level. Consequently, individual users of nursing models for research or practice may not need to explore the content of these two Areas. The steps given should be carefully reviewed by anyone considering implementation in a school of nursing, a nursing practice setting, a nursing service organization, and/or large research projects where groups will be involved in the implementation process. Sound organizational development principles and strategic planning approaches enhance implementation of any project, and will assist anyone desiring to implement a nursing model where more than one person is involved.

Area VI should be considered by all model users. Evaluation of actions taken, whether for a single project or for systematic implementation on an organizational level, should not be ignored. Evaluation checkpoints or processes designed prior to implementation will assist users in determining potential problem areas for early resolution thus preventing disruption of the overall model implementation; for example, use of a pilot project.

Although initially the steps and approaches suggested in this blueprint may seem overly structured, we believe that nursing models will be successfully implemented when care is taken in following the blueprint in education, practice, administration, and research.

THE BLUEPRINT

Area I. Exploration of the philosophical underpinnings of the model in question and the needs/philosophy of the setting/user.

  A. Critical questions for determining the fit of the conceptual model to the setting:
    1. What are the theoretical underpinnings of the proposed model(s)?

a. Many of the models are built on concepts and theories from physical, biological, social, and behavioral sciences. These may include stress and coping, group, general systems, and growth and development, to name a few.

2. What is the purpose of the model? Does it relate to the purpose and function planned for the use of the model?

3. What are the concepts and subconcepts? Are these concepts consistent with the philosophical approach and/or functional plan for use of the nursing model?

4. How are the concepts defined and what is the relationship among the concepts? Can their definition and relationship be easily transferred into the political and cultural environment of the setting?

5. What is the structure of the model? How does it relate to the view of nursing practice, education, research, or administration in the setting where use of the model is proposed?

6. What are the model's underlying assumptions? Can they be accepted or agreed on among the major players in the setting/organization planning to adopt a nursing model as an organizing framework?

Area II. Concept analysis of the proposed model, with important features defined for use in the setting/situation/organization.

Area III. Exploration of the more practical aspects of a particular model and its fit with the setting/situation/organization/project considering the adoption of a particular nursing model.

A. Critical questions related to practical application and potential implementation:

1. What is the purpose of the model? Will its purposes meet the need of the organization or project being considered?

2. What client or patient population will it address? Is there a fit with the purpose and population of the setting/situation/project where the model is to be implemented?

a. Individual

b. Family

    c. Group

    d. Community

3. How clear is the model? How difficult will it be for teaching and training of personnel, fellow practitioners, and/or researchers in the group?

4. Is the language used in the model consistent with the level of functioning and expertise in the setting/situation? What steps need to be taken to introduce/educate those using the model in this setting, situation, or project?

5. How simple or how complex is the model? How will this characteristic impact its acceptance or feasibility for teaching/training/research?

6. How general is the model? How accessible are experts to facilitate its effective adoption?

7. What is the feasibility of adopting/using the model, in terms of time, cost, and personnel training factors?

Area IV. Application of the principles of organizational development and a model for managed change as a guide for implementation of a nursing model (adapted from Tichy, 1991).

A. Step One: Assess the Setting/Situation/Organization (where the model is to be implemented).

1. What are the characteristics of communication within the organization?

2. What are the characteristics of decision making and how will they impact the acceptance/rejection of the use of a nursing model?

B. Step Two: Conduct a Diagnostic Plan. (This section will identify important questions and suggest methods of collecting data for decision making.)

1. What is the history of the organization? Are there any precluding factors that would prohibit adoption of a particular model?

2. What is the environment of the setting/organization/situation? Are there interdependencies or interrelationships that would facilitate or preclude adoption of a particular model?

    3. What resources are available? Are training and develop-
ment of forms for documentation required?

    4. Is the mission statement consistent or congruent with the
purpose and philosophy of the proposed model?

    5. What are the perceived goals? Is there goal congruence or
goal conflict with the adoption of a proposed model?

C. Step Three: Conduct an Analysis of Tasks and Competence.

    1. What basic tasks are needed to implement a nursing
model? By whom and for whom must these tasks be
performed?

    2. What is the nature of each task? What expertise is required?

    3. Can tasks be standardized in the setting/situation/
organization?

    4. What are the interrelationships among the tasks? Are com-
ponents of the tasks required under the span of control of
the person/organization planning to adopt a nursing
model?

D. Step Four: Conduct an Analysis of the People.

    1. What education and skill levels of personnel are needed for
this implementation? Are they consistent with the needs
for implementation of a nursing model?

    2. What are the expected personal characteristics of the
personnel (sex, age, risk taking, perseverance, positive
attitude)?

    3. What are the motivational forces that drive various partici-
pants in the process of adopting a model?

    4. What management personnel and technology will be
needed to implement this model?

    5. What is the perceived match between the proposed model
and what personnel involved in the process value as important? How does this valuation relate to the use of a nursing model?

Area V. Apply a strategic planning process for effective implementation for the use of a nursing model.

A. Steps in the Strategic Planning Process:

    1. Review and/or define the mission/purpose of use of a
nursing model in the setting/situation/organization.

2. Establish clear and achievable objectives.
    a. What are the short-range achievable objectives?
    b. What are the long-range objectives and outputs?
3. Develop a strategy for moving forward—a "road map."
    a. What is the time line? What is the relationship among tasks, training, and other factors for success?
4. Address the tactics of implementation.
    a. Has the operational planning included detailed specifications of who will do what, when, and how?
    b. Can the necessary resources (people, technical and financial) be obtained and utilized?
    c. Are there concrete plans for each step, function, group depending on the organization, and/or purpose of the use of the model?
5. Establish controls or monitoring methods that will guarantee that the tactics and time line are followed.
    a. Has the element included control various forms of monitoring:
        1. Tasks?
        2. Skills/Training?
        3. Financial resource use?
        4. Other aspects, depending on situation/purpose?
    b. What factors for success have become evident in the monitoring process?

Area VI. Plan and initiate evaluation processes and a system that is relevant to the purpose and goals for use of the model in the setting/situation/organization and/or project.

REFERENCES

Fawcett, J. (1989). *Analysis and evaluation of conceptual models of nursing* (2nd ed.). Philadelphia: Davis.

Leddy S., & Pepper, J. M. (1993). *Conceptual bases of professional nursing* (3rd ed.). Philadelphia: Lippincott.

Meleis, A. I. (1991). *Theoretical nursing: Development and progress* (2nd ed.). Philadelphia: Lippincott.

Meleis, A. I. (1995). Theory testing and theory support: Principles, challenges, and a sojourn into the future. In B. Neuman (Ed.), *The Neuman Systems Model* (3rd ed.). Norwalk, CT: Appleton & Lange.

Oermann, M. H. (Ed.). (1991). *Professional nursing practice: A conceptual approach.* Philadelphia: Lippincott.

Tichy, N. M. (1991). *Managing strategic change: Technical, political, and cultural dynamics.* New York: John Wiley & Sons.

2

Blueprint Example: An Integrated Model for Evaluation, Research, and Policy Analysis in the Context of Managed Care

Patricia Hinton Walker

*T*his chapter provides an example of how the *Blueprint* can be used to guide the process of selection and implementation of a conceptual model. To emphasize the relevance of nursing models to current and future practice and research, an "integrated model" has been selected for demonstration. The rationale for selection of this integrated conceptual model is actually found in the concluding chapter of this book, where Afaf Meleis identifies critical futuristic issues that must be addressed if nursing models are to be relevant in the 21st century. Meleis suggests "opening up extant theories for modifications, alterations, and further development."

The present chapter describes the development and implementation of the Neuman–Gil Model for Evaluation, Research, and Policy Analysis as an *example* based on the blueprint delineated in Chapter 1. This integrative model builds on the Neuman Systems Model and blends it with David Gil's model for social policy analysis (see Figure 2–1).

The model addresses some of the issues identified by Meleis in the concluding chapter, for example, the need for context-relevant theories and the development of integrative models that are applicable to new interdisciplinary practice roles and address broader goals for health and wellness in a global society (see Chapter 13). Other futuristic recommendations mentioned by Meleis that must be addressed through the use of nursing theoretical frameworks in the 21st century include: "theories for transitions," which address care within the community and across the continuum; "theories for global nursing care," which move beyond health status and address broader issues such as empowerment; and theories dealing with risks and costs of care in an environment where resources are shrinking.

The Neuman–Gil Model for Research, Evaluation, and Policy Analysis not only addresses Meleis's recommendations for the future but encourages users of other nursing models to expand their thinking and explore new ways of using nursing models. The purpose of this new integrative Neuman–Gil model is to guide research related to interdisciplinary care in community-based settings with a variety of populations in the context of managed care (Walker, 1991). Additionally, matching the *Blueprint* to an integrative model will guide users through the process of selecting and blending theoretical models from other disciplines with nursing, in order to address emerging issues associated with change in a global environment, such as population-based care, costs and quality outcomes of care, societal concerns in underserved communities, and other important policy-related issues.

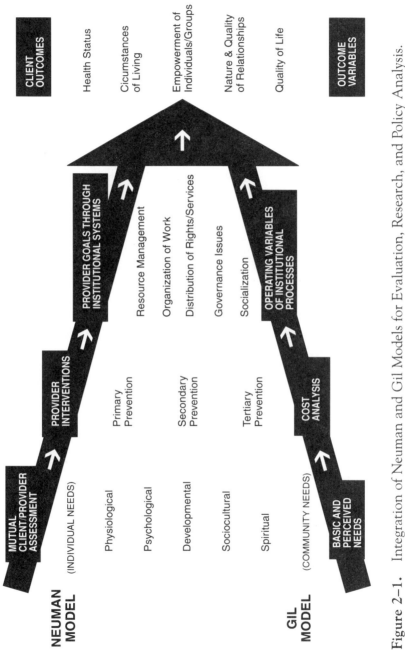

Figure 2–1. Integration of Neuman and Gil Models for Evaluation, Research, and Policy Analysis. Reprinted with permission of the University of Rochester Board of Trustees, 1994.

BACKGROUND

During the development of the University of Rochester School of Nursing Community Nursing Center (CNC), one significant challenge was to influence various satellite faculty practices by using a nursing theoretical framework in a new "nursing center without walls." Barrett (1993) has emphasized the importance of the use of nursing frameworks for developing nursing centers. She believes that "nursing centers should be guided by a philosophy and theoretical perspective always recognizable as nursing" (p. 15). She further believes that "nursing-science-based centers provide an opportunity for nursing to become the hub of the wheel of a new health care delivery system" (p. 16). Like Barrett, this author was particularly concerned about the need for the presence of scientific nursing in the development of scholarly practice and research in the CNC. This perspective is consistent with Fawcett's (1983) statement: "The importance of using conceptual models of nursing as guides for nursing research needs to be emphasized. ... . Thus their use can increase researchers' confidence that what they are doing is nursing research—not research in another discipline such as medicine, psychology, or sociology" (p. 171). Another significant goal for the CNC was to increase the influence of nursing theory-related practice and research in the education of students in the community. Clarke and Cody (1994) strongly support the linkage of current nursing practice, research, and education to nursing theoretical models: "Academicians and nursing leaders must overcome powerful barriers holding back radical change. The future of the nursing profession requires nursing theory-based education set in, and taught in, the homes, streets, and communities where people actually live their health" (p. 52).

In selecting and implementing a nursing theoretical model for the CNC, four challenges were evident:

1. How to use a nursing scientific framework to enhance the development of scholarly interdisciplinary practice in an academic environment.
2. How to influence student learning related to theoretical nursing approaches.

3. How to develop research to evaluate the contribution of advanced practice nursing in a variety of urban and rural settings from a common framework linking theoretical nursing.
4. How to link (a) research, (b) assessment of risk of populations, and (c) evaluation of cost and quality outcomes of care provided by advanced practice nurses in interdisciplinary practice roles, to health policy analysis.

The most difficult challenge was finding ways to link costs and economic variables to a nursing model; this linkage was not evident in the nursing literature.

Many nursing centers have had difficulty surviving in a health care market that is driven by economic and regulatory pressures. The University of Rochester CNC was developed as an innovative faculty practice with three major components: (a) *health policy* impact in a rapidly changing health care environment, (b) *business functions* based on sound business principles, and (c) *interdisciplinary practice* with a focus on nurse-managed care (see Figure 2-2). These three components would guide the development of an integrated

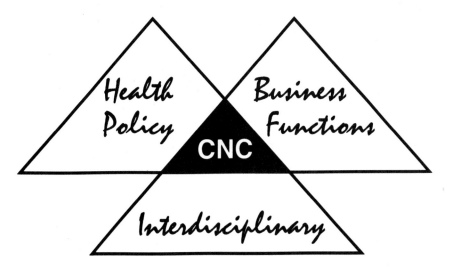

Figure 2–2. University of Rochester CNC Components for Success. Reprinted with permission of University of Rochester Board of Trustees, 1994.

model for practice, education, and research in the University of Rochester's unification environment, and would address financial and regulatory issues affecting practice.

It was important to consider the application and use of a nursing model and affirm the use of nursing frameworks in interdisciplinary practice and community-based care. Also, a sound conceptual research framework was needed to address the business and health policy issues—ideally, using a nursing model and testing its ability to provide structure and guidance to practice and research in this new nurse-managed organization. The business component of the model not only had to address the financial reimbursement and costing of care, but be adaptable to assess client satisfaction as an outcome of care. Could a nursing model qualify as the central core in an integrated model supporting business, health policy, and interdisciplinary practice? Instead of "testing" a nursing model, this author's approach was more consistent with the term "theory support," which Meleis (1995, p. 455) used to make the case for advocacy and evaluation of a particular nursing theory's potential and capability.

The result was the development of the Neuman–Gil integrative model to address emerging issues in this new and innovative approach to providing community-based care. Since its inception, the Neuman–Gil model has provided the conceptual framework for two studies: a pilot study of cost and quality outcomes of community-based care versus hospital care (freestanding birthing center study), and a survey sponsored and funded by the National Academies of Practice to determine similarities and differences among nine disciplines (dentistry, medicine, nursing, social work, psychology, optometry, osteopathic medicine, podiatry, and veterinary medicine) in assessment, interventions, and outcomes of care. The model breadth and flexibility might lend itself as a model of choice for interdisciplinary practice.

When considering modification and/or expansion of extant nursing models, an important challenge is not only to determine the fit of the nursing model to the situation/project/population, but also to explore the conceptual fit of models from other disciplines to the orientation of theoretical nursing. Some nurses might question the attempt to fit a policy analysis model with nursing; however, Weiner and Vining (1989) state that "policy analysis is as much an art and a craft as a science" (p. 12). They further emphasize the application of basic skills in a reasonably consistent way, and the need for a realistic perspective on the role of government in society, in order to influence policy. Nursing is both an art and a science. As a science, there is a need to influence the role of governmental policy on nursing practice, and this author developed an integrative model linking nursing to policy analysis. Consequently, this chapter demonstrates how the *Blueprint* can be used to select and implement nursing models, and also addresses the challenge of developing and implementing integrative models for the future. The main Areas of the *Blueprint* are reproduced here. Critical questions and steps for these Areas can be found in Chapter 1.

THE BLUEPRINT: A GUIDE FOR SELECTION AND IMPLEMENTATION

Area I. Exploration of the philosophical underpinnings of the model in question and the needs/philosophy of the setting/user.

Area II. Concept analysis of the proposed model, with important features defined for use in the setting/situation/organization.

The following sections address the philosophical underpinnings, conceptual fit, and relationships involved in using the Neuman–Gil model for nursing practice, education, and research in a community-based practice organization (University of Rochester CNC). The fit of the Neuman Systems Model (NSM) is discussed, and then the fit of Gil's Model for Social Policy Analysis (GMSPA) for this setting and purpose is explored.

NEUMAN SYSTEMS MODEL

A number of issues related to practice had to be considered when selecting a nursing model for the CNC. With a variety of practice sites, and with populations in both urban and rural areas, a broad comprehensive model was needed. Among the other selection criteria mentioned were philosophical underpinnings and the relationship of the fit to the structure of the model. Two key philosophical underpinnings of the Neuman Systems Model (NSM) were specifically appropriate for use with this CNC: (a) a systems theory approach and (b) the value of mutual goal setting and decision making between provider and client. The structure of the model was consistent with the practice and research needs of this organization. A broad approach to assessment, including developmental, spiritual, and sociocultural interacting variables (in addition to the usual psychological and physiological assessment), is critical for holistic care (Neuman, 1995). Attention to these variables is critical for assessing risk of populations in order to determine the appropriate level of intervention and to project costs of care.

As nurse providers begin to take a more active role in the managed care market—for example, negotiating contracts and establishing costs/prices for care—proactive risk assessment of the populations to be served is critical. The five variables of the client system in the NSM assist in identifying the focus variables that determine health risk. For example, in the adolescent population, risk is expected to be related more to developmental and psychological variables; in the chronically ill population, the risks are more likely to be associated with the physiological variable. The major focus of risk assessment may need to be on the sociocultural variable for populations living in poverty in inner-city communities, regardless of age and developmental status. Attention to these client system variables is very important in the total quality management (TQM) process of assessing customer satisfaction as an outcome of care. The connection of the NSM to the TQM process and customer satisfaction has already been developed (Walker, 1995a).

The structure of the NSM model, which focuses on prevention as intervention (defined as three levels of intervention), was extremely critical to positioning the CNC for intervention across the continuum of care. This comprehensive intervention structure should allow the nursing model to be used as a guide to determine differences in cost among primary, secondary, and tertiary preventions as interventions. This capacity is especially important in the emerging health care environment, where major concerns are duplication, fragmentation, inequities, expensive, and inappropriate utilization of services. Because much of the care provided through the CNC by advanced practice nurses was either primary prevention (health promotion, screening, primary care), and/or tertiary prevention (management of chronically ill and elderly), the intervention structure was critical for studying processes of care within a costing framework (Walker, 1995b).

The major concepts of the NSM are fairly consistent with most nursing models. However, subconcepts related to stressors, interaction with the environment, and the focus on prevention as intervention were critical to the selection of a model. Nurses must identify stressors in the community; for example, safety and violence as barriers to access to care, which contribute to increased stress and health care costs. As mentioned previously, prevention as intervention across the continuum of care was critical to the expansion into a framework for costing community-based care within the managed care environment. Except for the outcome changes in health status related to the disease process or health condition, the NSM did not specifically address policy approaches to studying systems of care, or other outcomes that needed to be addressed in local and global communities. Consequently, this author began seeking an outcome- oriented conceptual approaches for health policy analysis to integrate with the NSM. The systems approaches of both Newman and Gil were proven compatible and complementary.

GIL'S MODEL FOR SOCIAL POLICY ANALYSIS

When searching for a model for health policy analysis, a review of the literature produced an important article by McPherson (1987), which led to study of David Gil's work at Brandeis University. Critical to the search for a model that could be integrated with the NSM was a philosophical fit with the nursing profession and a clearly defined approach to outcomes. McPherson (1987) explained that health care policy is one type of social policy, and identified Gil's work as relevant to nursing because of nursing's social policy approach. The philosophical match with the history and roots of the discipline of nursing is evident. Chin (1983) states that "the concept of *society and environment* is consistently viewed as a central concept to the discipline. . . . The primary role of society–environment is viewed as a critical interacting factor . . ." (pp. 397–398). Gil

(1990) provides linkages among social policy, human biology, and institutional (governmental) systems. Schottland, in the foreword of Gil's book, identifies unsolved societal problems such as "Child abuse, homelessness . . . crime and juvenile delinquency, drug abuse, housing shortages for poor and low-income families . . . the fragmented health and medical system with millions denied access to medical care" (p. ix). The nursing literature related to community-based care is filled with practice and research publications that focus on many of these same problems.

Gil's model and methodology of analysis of social policies can be integrated with nursing to address many current issues in the context of health care reform. His approach addresses theoretical, methodological, philosophical, and political levels of social policy analysis (1990, p. xvi). All of these levels are relevant to nursing, particularly at a time when nursing is developing new practice roles to meet the diverse needs of communities, while still struggling with regulatory, political, and financial barriers. Gil's approach is simple and easy to understand, yet comprehensive enough to address the complexities of our current social and political world. His model is clearly a systems model—it has inputs, processes, and outputs—making compatible and congruent, the philosophical and conceptual underpinnings of the NSM and the Gil Model for Social Policy Analysis (GMSPA). Gil's premise is that "a model of social policies should identify key variables of all social policies, facilitate analysis of social policies and policy systems and their consequences, and aid in development of alternative policies and policy systems" (p. 20). He sees the evolution of social policies driven by basic human needs, which include: "(a) biological-material, (b) social-psychological, (c) productive-creative, (d) security, (e) self-actualization, and (f) spiritual needs" (p. 25). Although the NSM is not needs-based, there is clear similarity between the client variables in the NSM (physiological, psychological, sociocultural, developmental, and spiritual) and the needs identified by Gil.

Next, Gil (1990) describes five societal institutional systems or processes through which social policies are implemented, and emphasizes the interdependence and interaction between and among these key operating variables. These systems are: "(a) development, management, and conservation of natural and human-created resources; (b) organization of work and production; (c) exchange and distribution of goods, services, rights, and responsibilities, (d) governance and legitimation, and (e) reproduction, socialization, and social control" (p. 25). These operational variables are applicable to many of the struggles of the nursing profession, particularly in the development of community nursing centers to provide care to underserved populations and address needs of communities. The relevance and appropriateness for implementation in the CNC are addressed more fully in the discussion of Area III of the *Blueprint.*

The last part of the structure of this social policy analysis model is the output or outcomes of policy development and/or analysis. One of the strengths of this policy analysis model is its attention to outcomes. Because many of the provider organizations, government agencies, and new managed care companies are paying close attention to outcomes, a policy analysis model without outcomes cannot effectively address the need for policy changes. The outcomes identified by Gil (1990) are: "(a) circumstances of living of individuals, groups, and classes; (b) power of individuals, groups, and classes; (c) nature and quality of human relations among individuals, groups, and classes; and (d) overall quality of life" (p. 25). In addition to positive changes in health status, these outcomes are very consistent with interventions of advanced-practice nurses in community-based care settings. Consequently, the values, philosophical underpinnings, structure, and processes of this model are congruent not only with the profession of nursing but also with the Neuman Systems Model (NSM).

Area III. Exploration of the more practical aspects of a particular model and its fit with the setting/situation/organization/project considering the adoption of a particular nursing model.

In Area III of the *Blueprint,* questions related to the purpose of the model, populations served, language, and ease of teaching/ training personnel are posed. Again, the Neuman Systems Model (NSM) will be addressed first, followed by a discussion of its relevance to the Gil Model for Social Policy Analysis (GMSPA). Because the CNC is a community-based care organization, the nursing model selected and implemented needed to address *client* beyond the individual level. The NSM views the client system as an individual, a family, a group and/or a community (Walker, 1992). The nursing literature has provided practitioners with guidance for care (assessment and intervention) with families, groups, and communities in both national and international contexts. In the United States, where emphasis is on community and population-based care in the context of managed care, this was an important consideration. The target population and client focus of the model made it a good fit for this CNC multi-site practices.

A second consideration is easy comprehension of the language and an ability to teach/train personnel and/or incorporate other disciplines in the use of the model. In the context of CNC's partnerships with other interdisciplinary providers and community groups, evaluation of the language of the model was significant. The consumer-sensitive terminology of this model is an important consideration for these partnerships and future international consultation (Walker, 1991). Because most providers and laypersons can relate to stressors, environment, prevention, and lines of defense, this model is easy to teach and use with other groups outside nursing. Time, cost implications, and access to experts were not barriers to implementing this integrated model. (This advantage is discussed more specifically under Areas IV and V of the *Blueprint.*)

From a practical perspective, the GMSPA was clearly applicable to this purpose and setting. Gil's approach to analysis of the client or client population was both conceptually and operationally similar to that of the NSM and was easy to integrate into the NSM holistic approach. Additionally, the operational variables and outcomes of his model were especially valuable in the development of the CNC approach to evaluation, research, and policy analysis. Regarding the barriers to community-based care provided by advanced-practice nurses, the institutional systems/processes help address reasons for existence in the community as well as barriers to care of populations and rights to practice. A detailed explanation of the applicability of the GMSPA and its integration with the NSM answers many of the questions posed in Area III of the *Blueprint.*

The five institutional systems or processes identified by Gil (1990) were referenced previously. When considering the use of Gil's model for the CNC, the five societal institutional processes or operating variables (referenced earlier) were appropriate to both the mission and the barriers experienced by advanced-practice nurses and to the survival of nursing centers. The first operating variable was identified as "development, management, and conservation of natural and human-created resources." In the context of development of community-based care, the creative development and management of resources was a key not only to successful partnerships with the community, but also to sound business practices. The philosophy of the CNC was to build on current resources in the community and to work through partnerships for resources, including: practice sites (buildings); collaborative arrangements for billing, to reduce costs; and enlistment of community-supported volunteers for receptions and similar functions. At the heart of the success of most nursing centers in the country is the joint use and management of community resources for both financial and partnership success. In the University of Rochester CNC, this arrangement described practices at a troubled home for teens, a neighborhood center in partnership with the Sisters of St. Joseph, a school-based clinic, and many rural contracts and primary care practices.

A second operating variable related to the "organization of work and production" (Gil, 1990). This variable was very important to the development and evaluation of what is called in the literature *nurse-managed care*. The production of health care and the traditional organization of work supporting this societal function in the United States have fulfilled the medical model of care, delivered and controlled by physicians. Part of the nursing challenge, particularly in research, is to demonstrate the value of community-based care managed or "produced" by nurses to underserved populations. Although nurses know and recognize that nurse-managed care is truly a form of interdisciplinary care, our profession has not conducted sufficient research to support the change in the traditional "organization of work" for health care in this country. The recent move toward managed care seems to be addressing Conway's (1983) points that "greater support of interdisciplinary research in primary care may well become a government priority as a matter of policy to implement the government's publicly stated intentions to bring about a higher level of personal health for an increased portion of the population" (p. 35). It was this author's belief that nursing leaders, particularly those involved with community-based nurse-managed care should be prepared to address these needs from a sound conceptual approach.

The third operating variable or institutional process actually relates both to the rights and privileges of the populations served by nursing and to those of the nursing profession. The "exchange and distribution of goods, services, rights, and responsibilities" (Gil, 1990) for our patients and clients clearly refers to problems in the distribution of health care and the lack of access to care experienced by many underserved populations. The key reason for the existence of many nursing centers is this lack of distribution of services and rights to health care. This situation today traces its history to nursing centers such as the Henry Street Settlement, Margaret Sanger's birth control clinic, and the Frontier Nursing Service (Glass, 1989). Another aspect of this operating variable relates to the rights of nurses. It is not the purpose of this chapter to discuss in detail how nurses' rights and services have been limited, but the nursing literature is filled with references about limitations specifically placed on prescriptive privileges, rights to practice, and reimbursement (Walker, 1994). The relationship between the limited rights of certain urban and rural populations to access to care, and the limited rights of nurses to practice and be reimbursed for care provided, is significant for health policy analysis and relevant to this variable. Nurses must continue to influence institutional (governmental) systems with scientifically valid practice and research data in order to best impact changes in health policy.

The last two operating variables are clearly related to the previous discussion: "governance and legitimation" and "reproduction, socialization, and social control" (Gil, 1990). Unfortunately, issues of governance and legitimation related to access, distribution, and financial control of health care systems and dollars in the United States are caught in the political process. Questions in political debates center around the future survival or demise of many social policies, particularly those related to underserved populations. The nursing profession must understand, articulate, and better support (through research results) the relationship between economic and social forces in order to impact future policy. We not only have a "socialization" challenge of educating legislators, health care consumers, and purchasers about the value of nursing, but we should do this with a clear understanding of the relationship between economic and social policy.

Outcomes of the GMSPA were a very important reason for choosing to integrate this model with a nursing model. Again, in the context of community-based care, many nurses have historically struggled with improvement of "circumstances of living of individuals, groups, and classes of people" (Gil, 1990). This outcome relates to assessment and evaluation of functional status and is applicable to nurse-managed care of: homeless populations, victims of violence in communities, children and families in public housing settings, elderly populations in group or private homes, and basic nursing care of the disabled and the chronically ill. Also, the nursing role of patient- and consumer-advocate is also consistent with "empowerment of individuals, groups, and classes of people" as an important outcome of care. This is particularly evident in the nursing literature related to care of women, teens, and underserved populations, and maternal-child care given by midwives. Evaluation of nursing's focus on family-centered care of women, children, troubled teenagers, chronically ill populations, and the elderly can be measured under Gil's third outcome "nature and quality of human relationships among individuals, groups, and classes" (Gil, 1990). Last, changes in "overall quality of life" are a goal or outcome of nursing care with patients/clients/consumers of all ages, particularly the chronically ill, terminally ill, and elderly. This author believes that the Gil model, integrated with a nursing model, can provide a framework within which we can study and document policy-related issues.

Because the Gil model was not specifically designed for just "health," the outcome of health status was added to these outcomes for the integrated Neuman–Gil Model (see Figure 2–1). In the context of today's managed care environment, nursing's contribution to quality of care must be clearly demonstrated. To impact policies of government and business, the two largest purchasers of health care, nurses must conduct health services research that documents either equivalent or better improvement of health status related to specific conditions. It is not this author's intent to say that nursing care is better than physician care, but nurses must at least document statistically equivalent quality of care measured in clinical outcomes at lower costs, in order to influence health care and reimbursement policy. This integrative model clearly fits the mission, goals, and purposes of organizations interested in quality and cost-effective community-based care across the continuum.

Area IV. Application of the principles of organizational development and a model for managed change as a guide for implementation of a nursing model.

Area V. Application of strategic planning process for effective implementation of the use of a nursing model.

Areas IV and V will be addressed briefly, without specific attention to each Area. In the development of the CNC and the adaptation of conceptual models, strategic planning processes were used. There was congruence between the mission of the CNC organization and the Neuman–Gil Model. There was also consistency with the goals of the CNC advanced-practice nursing faculty. These goals included: contributing to the profession through scholarship in practice and research; survival in these new practice sites from a business/financial perspective; and nurses' influence on health policy at local, state, and federal levels. Most importantly, the fit of the models with the purpose and setting facilitated the actual implementation.

From an organizational and structural standpoint, the CNC was designed as a separate practice corporation connected to the School of Nursing. Decision making among the School of Nursing faculty as a whole was not a problem. In many ways, the CNC as a care-provider organization is similar to the nearby hospital system (Strong Memorial Hospital), along with the School of Medicine and School of Nursing, is part of the University of Rochester Medical Center. The CNC was considered as a site for education of students, faculty practice, and an evolving research program. The CNC clinical faculty were consulted, and they found the model consistent with the overall CNC approach. Many of the faculty needed scholarly presentations/publications for promotion, and they subsequently published articles and chapters about their CNC practice in the context of these conceptual models.

In this faculty practice model, education of the users was not a problem because the model was used to guide practice in a general and conceptual way. However, as systems are being developed to track outcomes of CNC clients in some settings, considerations about instrument development and information systems reflecting assessment, processes, and outcomes of care related to the Neuman–Gil Model are currently being explored. The language and commonsense approach of both original models make them easy to understand or translate, so this aspect of model use does not pose a barrier to implementation. There were, however, considerations related to language when the Neuman–Gil Model was implemented as a framework for the interdisciplinary survey with the National Academies of Practice (NAP). Some terms from the Neuman Systems Model were objectionable to physician colleagues in the NAP survey; for example, "holistic" was replaced by "comprehensive" for the purposes of the survey. Also, the term "provider" was used to replace "nurse" (usually associated with the NSM). However, language related to the levels of intervention (NSM) and the outcomes of care (GMSPA) were familiar to the different disciplines and acceptable for use in the survey.

The Neuman–Gil Model is being used as a framework to guide evaluation and research in the CNC. A pilot study comparing cost and quality outcomes of a freestanding birthing center (primary prevention) with traditional OB care and hospital delivery (secondary prevention) is currently being presented and published. Study results indicate that the primary prevention model was less interventive and less costly, with no significant difference in the clinical outcomes for mothers and babies. This integrative model is also being used to guide selection of instruments and customization of data systems for a school-based health center in Rochester, New York. However, for the purposes of this chapter, the implementation related to the interdisciplinary survey with the NAP will be described.

A presentation at a National Academies of Practice (NAP) conference, which highlighted interdisciplinary roles in the context of community-based care, created the interest for a survey using the Neuman–Gil Model. Because one of the goals and objectives of the NAP is to support and evaluate the impact of interdisciplinary practice, the NAP Council funded a survey of the nine disciplines mentioned earlier, to determine similarities and differences among disciplines using the Neuman–Gil Model. This was seen as the first step of a long-range objective for the NAP: to more clearly articulate the value of interdisciplinary practice in the context of managed care. The survey was piloted through the governing council, where a few changes were made, specifically those related to language and terms within the NSM, such as "holistic" care. Resources were obtained through the NAP's funding of the project, and two mailings of the survey were subsequently completed. Response rate averaged 51.6% across the nine disciplines. Sound research controls were put into place to prevent duplication of responses between the first and second mailings, and to clearly document responses from the different disciplines. Results from this survey, using the Neuman–Gil Model, are being analyzed at the time of this writing.

Area VI. Plan and initiate evaluation processes and a system that is relevant to the purpose and goals for use of the model in the setting/situation/organization and/or project.

Evaluation of the effectiveness of the Neuman–Gil Model is ongoing. Some of the strategies and processes planned include:

1. Feedback of perceived value and utility by other disciplines as a framework for practice, education, and research.
2. Demonstration of the value of this model for externally funded practice-based research projects.
3. Opportunities to inform policy and other disciplines (including economists) outside the nursing profession through publication, presentation of data using the model, and use by professional organizations to influence legislators.
4. Feedback from the nursing profession related to the value of the model, measured by requests for information, consultation, and publication reprints about the Neuman–Gil Model.

Although this integrative model is still very new, based on the response to presentations about its use, the number of requests for information about its value and use will continue to increase.

REFERENCES

Barrett, E. M. (1993, Fall). Nursing centers without nursing frameworks: What's wrong with this picture? *Nursing Science Quarterly.*

Chin, P. L. (1983). Nursing theory development: Where we have been and where we are going. In N. L. Chaska (Ed.), *The nursing profession: A time to speak.* New York: McGraw-Hill.

Clarke, P. N., & Cody, W. K. (1994). Nursing theory-based practice in the home and community: The crux of professional nursing education. *Advances in Nursing Science, 17*(2), 41–53.

Conway, M. E. (1983). Prescription for professionalization. In N. L. Chaska (Ed.), *The nursing profession: A time to speak.* New York: McGraw-Hill.

Fawcett, J. (1983). Contemporary nursing research: Its relevance for nursing practice. In N. L. Chaska (Ed.), *The nursing profession: A time to speak.* New York: McGraw-Hill.

Gil, D. G. (1990). *Unraveling social policy: Theory, analysis, and political action towards social equality* (4th ed.). Rochester, VT: Schenkman Books.

Glass, L. K. (1989). The historic origins of nursing centers. In *Nursing centers: Meeting the demand for quality health care.* New York: National League for Nursing.

McPherson, K. M. (1987). Health care policy, values, and nursing. *Advances in Nursing Science, 9*(3), 1–11.

Meleis, A. I. (1991). *Theoretical nursing: Development and progress* (2nd ed.). Philadelphia: Lippincott.

Meleis, A. I. (1995). Theory testing and theory support: Principles, challenges, and a sojourn into the future. In B. Neuman (Ed.), *The Neuman Systems Model* (3rd ed.). Norwalk, CT: Appleton & Lange.

Neuman, B. (1995). The Neuman Systems Model. In B. Neuman (Ed.), *The Neuman Systems Model* (3rd ed.). Norwalk, CT: Appleton & Lange.

Walker, P. H. (1991, Fall). The community nursing center for nurse practitioners: An opportunity to develop entrepreneurial skills. *Rochester Nursing,* 18, 19, 19–21.

Walker, P. H. (1992). Neuman Systems Model: Right choice for community nursing center. *Neuman News, 3*(1), 1–2.

Walker, P. H. (1994). Dollars and sense in health reform: Interdisciplinary practice and community nursing centers. *Nursing Administration Quarterly, 19*(1), 1–11.

Walker, P. H. (1995a). TQM and the Neuman Systems Model: Education for health care administration. In B. Neuman (Ed.), *The Neuman Systems Model* (3rd ed., pp. 365–376). Norwalk, CT: Appleton & Lange.

Walker, P. H. (1995b). Neuman-based education, practice, and research in a community nursing center. In B. Neuman (Ed.), *The Neuman Systems Model* (3rd ed., pp. 415–442). Norwalk, CT: Appleton & Lange.

Weiner, D. L., & Vining, A. R. (1989). *Policy analysis: Concepts and practice.* Englewood Cliffs, NJ: Prentice-Hall.

Section II

Blueprints for Research

3

The Johnson Behavioral System Model: Explaining Activities of Chronically Ill Children

Bonnie Holaday, Anne Turner-Henson, and James Swan

The scholar using the behavioral system model for nursing has two major foci in developing nursing science. Problems in the structure or function of the behavioral system and its subsystems are one focus. The task is to identify, describe, and explain these problems. The other focus is the prevention and treatment of these problems. In this instance, the task is to develop the scientific bases for

This work was supported by Grant MCJ06550 from the Maternal Child Health Program (Title V, Social Security Act), Health Resources and Services Administration, Department of Health and Human Resources, and by Grant NU 01374, National Center for Nursing Research, National Institutes of Health.

intervention as well as specific methodologies for doing so. Holaday and her as-
sociates pay greater attention in this paper to the first of these foci, but they
clearly have not forgotten the other. Through Holaday's long series of studies of
achievement behavior in chronically ill children, she has used both foci to begin
building a body of knowledge in this area. Her work, and that of her colleagues,
exemplifies quite well the value of cumulative research in the development of a
sound substantive base in a practice field.

Dorothy E. Johnson

---

*I*n this chapter, we explore the application of the Johnson Behavioral System (JBS) Model (Johnson 1980, 1990) to a research project
directed toward explaining activity patterns of chronically ill
school-age children. The project's goal was to determine the influence of *sustenal* imperatives—protection, nurturance, and stimulation—on activity patterns. The JBS Model posits that human beings
meet life demands through behavioral balance achieved from the
structural integrity and function of six subsystems:

1. Achievement.
2. Affiliative.
3. Aggressive/Protective Dependence.
4. Eliminative.
5. Ingestive.
6. Sexual.

Faculty and clinicians working with the model added Restorative to
the list of subsystems (Auger, 1976). For these subsystems to develop and maintain stability, each must have a constant supply of
functional requirements.

VARIABLES THAT INFLUENCE
CHILDREN'S ACTIVITIES

The term "variable" is synonymous with the concept of environment; it encompasses factors that are outside the boundary of the

behavioral system but have the capacity to alter or change behavior within the system. Variables are the source from which the individual draws the susternal imperatives (see Figure 3–1) that provide the prerequisites for maintaining healthy behavior. A detailed description of sustenal imperatives is provided in Grubbs's (1980) seminal article.

Over time, an examination of patterns of children's activities provides a great deal of information about the changing conditions of

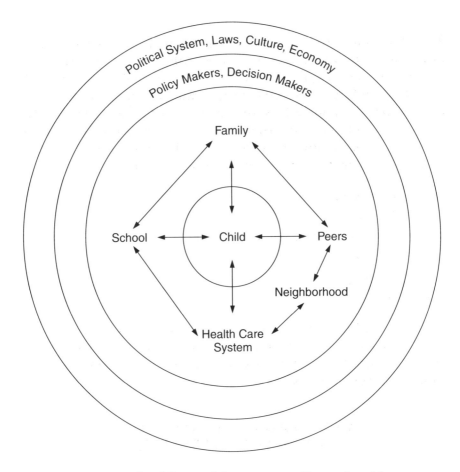

Figure 3–1. Supply of Sustenal Imperatives—Protection, Nurturance, and Stimulation.

childhood in society, childbearing beliefs and practices, and how society prepares children for adulthood (Medrich, Roizen, Rubin, & Buckley, 1982). Everyday life experiences, including physical and nonphysical activities, provide opportunities for children's development and socialization. Childhood is a time of independence and exploration in preparation for adulthood; during these developmental years, activity patterns are shaped and learned. How children spend their time—their selection of activities—may be considered a proxy for their interests; an indicator of what matters to them and to their families and peers; and a measure of their abilities and of the opportunities and constraints present within their environments.

Although we know a great deal about the influences on healthy children's activities, little is known about the influences that impact chronically ill children's activities. Chronically ill children have long been considered at risk for psychosocial morbidity (Cadman, Boyle, & Szatmari, 1987; Weiland, Pless, & Roughman, 1992). Studies have noted that these children may have significantly more psychosocial difficulties, evidenced as behavioral, social, and school problems (Larigne & Faier-Routman, 1992; Pless, Power, & Peckham, 1993) that potentially impact their activities. The children's participation in activities may also be influenced by restrictions in day-to-day experiences, interpersonal communication, mobility, self-care or treatment, and endurance. From a behavioral systems approach, several variables can be identified as influencing children's activities. These variables—personal physiology, family, peers, and the health care system—exert a strong influence over the types of activities in which children engage. Therefore, through an understanding of the influence of variables that shape chronically ill children's activities, one may address the variables that adversely affect the chronically ill child's ability to interact and grow through these experiences.

Physiological

Activity is beneficial not only to children's psychomotor development, but also to their physiological subsystems. Among American children, cardiovascular disease risk factors are appearing early in childhood in an alarming rate (Drake & Kuntzleman, 1988). An increasing incidence of obesity (Gortmaker, Dietz, & Cheung, 1990), a 10% decline in aerobic fitness (Updyke & Willett, 1989), and a disturbing trend of decreasing physical activity with age all contribute to an increasing frequency of sedentary lifestyle among American children. The physiological benefits of physical activity have been well documented in healthy children and, to some extent, from a primarily physiological perspective, in children with specific chronic illnesses. However, the long-term benefits and the behavioral components of prolonged physical activity are not well understood.

The physiological benefits of activity have been documented in chronically ill children from a disease-specific perspective rather than from a noncategorical perspective. Improvement in glycemic control, with a resulting reduction in long-term complications related to diabetes, has been documented in children with Type 1 diabetes (Campaigne, Gilliam, & Spencer, 1984; Dorchy & Poortman, 1989). Improvements in motor ability and flexibility have been documented in children with cerebral palsy (Bar-Or, Inbar, & Spira, 1976) and in children with other neuromuscular disorders.

In children with respiratory disorders, physiological benefits have been well researched. In children with asthma, the most common form of chronic illness in childhood, a sedentary lifestyle, compounded by poor physical fitness, has been directly associated with poor asthma control. Physical fitness programs that focus on aerobic fitness and reduction of sedentary lifestyle have been found to be beneficial not only to overall fitness (both cardiovascular and endurance), but also to asthma control (Fink, Kaye, Blau, & Spiter, 1993; Goldberg, 1990; Orenstein, Reed, Grogan, & Crawford, 1985). In children with cystic fibrosis, short-term studies about aerobic exercise have documented improvements in cardiovascular fitness, exercise tolerance, and possible improvement in lung functioning or delay in the expected lung deterioration characteristic of the disease's progression (Orenstein et al., 1985). Few studies have explored the relationship between physiological and behavioral factors and children's activities, although it is well documented that motivation and skills are needed to lay the foundation for a physically active lifestyle (Sallis et al., 1992). Alongside the focus on normal children's activities and fitness, there is minimal information about these concerns in children with chronic illness (Bar-Or, 1990; Challenor, 1989), and very few studies have been directed toward identifying the determinants of low activity patterns and low levels of physical fitness in children with chronic illness.

Family

The importance of the amount and quality of time parents spend on their children's development has been well established, and research clearly links a lack of parental involvement with children with poor developmental outcomes. Conditions for families are strained today by increased family mobility (U.S. Bureau of the Census, 1995), smaller family size (U.S. Bureau of the Census, 1995), increased number of families with both parents in the workforce (U.S. Department of Labor, 1994), and increased number of families living in poverty (U.S. Bureau of the Census, 1995). Additionally, many families today lack the support of extended family members, have fewer siblings for in-home help, and must limit family opportunities for recreational time because of financial constraints. More mothers are raising children alone, and, in many families, both parents have out-of-home work demands and responsibilities.

For many families in America today, maternal employment is an economic necessity, although environmental support is often lacking (Bronfenbrenner, 1986). Resources such as schools, parks, recreation programs, after-school day care, and libraries are essential for families. For children whose mothers are employed, access to these resources is essential for opportunities to socialize with peers. Thus, when parents' roles are strained by the multiple demands on their time (Hochschild, 1989), access to these resources reduces stress and promotes important socialization opportunities for the children.

Childrearing roles of parents and responsibilities of siblings in families with a chronically ill child are challenged by the increased demands and restrictions imposed by the illness. Families may experience the time-consuming burden of daily caregiving (Stevens, 1994; Turner-Henson, Holaday, & Swan, 1992); social isolation and lack of psychological support, which can lead to family dysfunction (Woods, Yates, & Primomo, 1984); and increased out-of-pocket health care expenditures, which can result in heavy financial burdens and lifelong debt (Brooten, Klein, Stringer, York, & Brown, 1993; Paterson, 1993). In addition, families with chronically ill children face numerous contacts with the health care system, altered plans for family outings and vacations, parental fatigue, and depression (Hobbs, Perrin, & Ireys, 1985; Jessop, Riesmann, & Stein, 1988; Marcenko & Meyers, 1991). Consequently, the important time that parents spend on activities with chronically ill children may be limited.

Regarding physical activity, the involvement of children appears to be related to parental encouragement in participation (Moore, Lombardi, White, Campbell, Oliveria, & Ellison, 1991; Ross & Pate, 1987; Sallis, Alcaraz, McKenzie, Hovell, Kolody, & Nader, 1992).

Peers

Peer relations are crucial to children's psychological and social development. Peer relations during childhood have been documented to be predictors of adjustment and competence during adolescence, and adaptation into adulthood (Burton & Krantz, 1990; Landau & Milich, 1990; Noll, Rio, Davies, Bukowski, & Koontz, 1992). Solitary children, or children without friends, experience loneliness and psychological distress about their circumstances (Crick & Ladd, 1993). Chronically ill children experience particular difficulties with peer interaction: social isolation (Cadman, Boyle, & Szatmari, 1987), peers' perceptions of poor social capabilities (Armstrong, Rosenbaum, & Kling, 1992), and strained rapport with peers (Streitmatter & Pate, 1989), all of which diminish these children's everyday life activities with peers.

Participation in organized activities enables children to shape cognitive, creative, and physical skills through meaningful group experiences (Medrich et al., 1982). Team sports, after-school lessons, and organized social groups allow children to participate in peer and prosocial behaviors in preparation for the adult world. For the chronically ill child, the important developmental task of practicing peer and prosocial behaviors through peer and social interactions may be compromised by a limited access to such activities.

Neighborhood

The neighborhood or community can play a critical role in supporting families, ameliorating isolation, promoting group values, and providing resources (Garbanino, 1985). Factors within the neighborhood, such as population density and economic and organizational resources, can greatly impact children's activities. Research has clearly documented the influence of these factors on healthy children's activities, but a projection of their impact or beneficial effect on chronically ill children's activities has little verification in the literature.

The neighborhood is one of the most influential settings, in terms of children's activities. The physical qualities of a neighborhood are important determinants of its resident children's spontaneity (Medrich et al., 1982; Noschis, 1992; Lennard & Lennard, 1992). High-population environments, such as inner-city or urban areas, may offer copious resources for stimulating and developmentally appropriate activities, (i.e., community parks, libraries, recreation centers), but issues of safety, cost, and accessibility may deter children's participation. Research has documented that such high-density neighborhoods, while stimulating for the emotional development of older children, tend to have a negative effect on the social and emotional development of younger children (Bronfenbrenner, 1986). On the other hand, low-density neighborhoods (e.g., rural areas) have been found to be associated with social isolation, limited resources, and fewer opportunities for stimulating activities for children, though safety issues are fewer, compared to higher-density settings (Rutenfranz, Anderson, Seliger, & Masironi, 1982). Suburban environments have been documented to be detrimental to school-age children's development in that they tend to provide fewer opportunities for the enhancement of competence (Hart, 1977; Weinstein & David, 1987).

When children's environments are enriched by the presence of facilities such as parks, recreation centers, libraries, community pools, and playgrounds, the impact on their ability to participate in activities is favorable.

Summary

Nurses using the JBS in research are interested in examining the factors or processes that put children at risk of not maintaining a behavioral system balance and, therefore, not developing to their full potential. Children who are not receiving adequate amounts of protection, nurturance, and stimulation from susternal imperatives can be classified as being at risk for an imbalanced behavioral system or a deficiency in desirable life experiences. The more risk factors in a child's life and the longer the periods of time during which those factors are present, the more likely the child will experience a behavioral system imbalance.

METHOD

The dependent variable in this study was *physical activities,* a component of the restorative subsystem (restorative to relieve fatigue and/or achieve a state of equilibrium by reestablishing or replenishing the energy distribution among other subsystems; to redistribute energy). Participation in physical activities may also lead to experiences of mastery (achievement), interaction with other children (affiliative), and clarification of gender identity (sexual). Physical activities, the variable area of interest, have been divided into different levels (0 = nonphysical; 1 to 4 = levels of activity, with 4 being the most active). The independent variables, the supply source from which the individual draws sustenal imperatives, are outlined in Table 3-3. Over time, variables may be internalized as regulating or control mechanisms so that they are no longer only outside the system. For example, a ten-year-old White female with asthma may internalize expectations and behaviors based on perceived societal norms. Because control mechanisms are internalized, they often must be inferred from behavior.

Design

A cross-sectional survey was used to collect data at one point in time from a sample of 10- to 12-year-old chronically ill children. The overall purpose of the study was to describe and analyze everyday life experiences through an examination of chronically ill children's use of time outside of school. A component of the study focused on children's views of physical activity.

Subjects

The sample consisted of 365 children with chronic illnesses. They were randomly selected from a sampling frame of 912 chronically ill children from the Standard Metropolitan Statistical Area (SMSA) of Birmingham (Alabama) (N = 156) and of San Francisco (N = 209). (A detailed discussion of the development of the sampling frame and subject selection is provided in Turner-Henson, Holaday, and O'Sullivan, (1992).)

The sample for the study consisted of 58% males (N = 209) and 42% females (N = 156). The majority were White (59%); Black (24%); Asian (5%); and Hispanic (4%) participants comprised the other major groups. The age distribution of the sample was 35% (N = 128) ten-year-olds; 25% (N = 90) eleven-year-olds; and 41% (N = 148) twelve-year-olds. For purposes of the analysis, social economic status (SES) was treated as a three-level variable: 31% (N = 113) low SES; 33% (N = 123) middle SES; and 35% (N = 129) high SES. Sixty-three percent of the mothers were employed, and 68% of the children resided in dual-parent households.

A chronic illness was defined as an impairment or deviation from normal that had one or more of the following characteristics: permanent; residual disability; cursed by nonreversible pathological attention; special training of the patient for rehabilitation; expected to require a long period of supervision or care (Mayo, 1956). A noncategorical approach (Stein & Jessop, 1989), focusing on commonalities across disease categories rather than on specific disease types (e.g., asthma versus diabetes), was used. This approach provided a wide range of diagnostic entities, resulting in a comprehensive representation of the experiences of chronically ill children. Many health professionals recognize that children with chronic disease share many needs in common, irrespective of what disease they may have (Hobbs, Perrin, & Ireys, 1985). All children in this study were diagnosed with chronic illnesses that did not affect communication, vision, hearing, intellectual ability, or school enrollment. The four most common diagnoses were asthma 25% (N = 91), congenital heart disease 18% (N = 66), neuromuscular disorder 15% (N = 54), and diabetes 14% (N = 50).

Procedure

Data were collected via a questionnaire battery administered by female interviewers in the children's homes. All interviewers were trained by the Survey Research Center, University of California, Berkeley. Consent to participate in the study was signed by the parent (or other primary caretaker) responsible for the child's time after school (in 93% of the cases, this was the mother or another female), and the child signed an assent form. After the parent/caretaker and child completed their questionnaires, the parent/caretaker was interviewed using a medical background questionnaire.

Measures

The child was interviewed using a 59-item open-ended and multiple-choice questionnaire. Chronically ill children were asked about their activities alone and with friends; a wide variety of activities, both physical and nonphysical, were considered. Table 3-1 lists the activities according to whether they were nonphysical (level 0) or involved varied degrees of physical activity (levels 1 to 4, with level 4 being the most active).

Indexes of numbers of reported activities were created for each item (alone and with friends), for physical and nonphysical activities, and for each level of physical activity. Overall indexes were also created: all physical activities, all nonphysical activities, all activities with friends, all activities alone, and all activities.

Test–retest, to check the stability of the children's responses to factual questions, demonstrated 90% agreement at two months postinterview (Holaday, Turner-Henson, & Swan, 1991). Details about questionnaire construction and validity are provided elsewhere (Holaday & Turner-Henson, 1989). The 83-item parent/caretaker questionnaire probed socialization priorities, childbearing practices, and questions about the neighborhood and available services. Parents were also given a mix of open-ended and multiple-choice questions. Test–retest of the parents' responses at two months postinterview found 98% agreement (Holaday, Turner-Henson, & Swan, 1991).

Table 3–1
Levels of Physical Activity

Level 0	no reported activity
	nonphysical activity reported:
	collections/toys
	found objects
	nurturing (pets, plants, etc.)
	construction (models, building, fixing, etc.)
	arts and crafts
	media (listen, watch, read, homework, computer)
	going places
	shopping
	board games
	socializing
	housework/chores
	personal care
Level 1	role-playing games
	playing/going outside
Level 2	baseball
	softball
	bowling
	gymnastics
	ping pong
	mini-biking/motorcycling
	dance
	tetherball
	playing catch/frisbee
Level 3	football
	kickball
	soccer
	other 1- or 2-person sports (e.g., wrestling, martial arts)
	sports, unspecified
Level 4	basketball
	volleyball
	other team sports
	roller skating
	skating, unspecified
	swimming
	tennis
	bicycling
	skateboarding
	camping/backpacking
	fishing/hunting
	hiking/walking
	horseback riding

Data Management

Management of data was directed by the Survey Research Center, University of California, Berkeley. Completed interviews were edited by the interviewer and then by the field supervisor. If necessary, follow-up phone calls were made to parents to complete unanswered questions or to clarify responses. Data were again edited, reduced, and coded by the Survey Research Center.

RESULTS

Overall, children reported about 2.5 activities with friends, the same number alone, and, accounting for duplication of the same activity with friends and alone, 4.6 overall (see Table 3–2). However, one-fourth reported engaging in no activities with friends, and all but 4 children reported activities alone. An average of about 2 activities were physical; four-fifths of them were done with friends and were more likely to be engaged in with friends than alone. By contrast, of an average of almost 3 nonphysical activities, two-thirds were done alone and were much less likely to be engaged in with friends than alone. This reproduces the pattern that Medrich and associates (1982) found for a general population of children.

The issue was: What home and individual factors affect children's participation, particularly in physical activities? Table 3–3 lists hypothetical explanations of such participation, outlining a number of patterns of expected influence. Parents' involvement in volunteer work touching on children's lives was expected to foster their children's involvement in all types of activities. Higher family income was expected to increase activities with friends and reduce those alone; caregiver education was predicted to increase physical and reduce nonphysical activities. Single-parent households were thought to foster nonphysical activities while reducing physical activities with friends; multiple-adult households were expected to discourage activities alone. Caregiver employment outside the home was expected to reduce all physical activities and to increase passive activities alone.

Table 3–2
Activities Reported by Chronically Ill Children (N = 365)

Measure	Mean	Standard Deviation	Percentage Engaged
Physical Activities			
With friends	1.55	1.39	67.9%
Alone	0.56	0.68	45.8
Either	1.93	1.47	80.3
Level 1	0.48	0.60	42.5
Level 2	0.28	0.50	25.2
Level 3	0.44	0.64	36.4
Level 4	0.74	0.84	51.5
Nonphysical Activities			
With friends	0.97	1.14	54.0
Alone	1.92	0.91	91.8
Either	2.69	1.44	96.7
All Activities			
With friends	2.52	1.77	74.0
Alone	2.48	0.74	98.9
Both	4.62	1.80	99.5
Physical Minus Nonphysical			
With friends	0.59	1.83	—
Alone	−1.36	1.43	—
Both	−0.78	2.53	—

Among the children, boys were expected to engage in more physical but fewer nonphysical activities than girls. Older children in the study were expected to engage in fewer physical activities, as undifferentiated physical play became replaced with more specialized, organized physical activities. Seriousness of illness was expected to reduce all activities other than passive activities alone, which severe illness was predicted to foster. Having more playmates was hypothesized to be related to more activities with friends and to fewer passive activities alone.

To examine the impact of neighborhood activities on the children's development, the study used Bryant's (1985) concept that people, places, and activities in a neighborhood provide opportunities and interpersonal support to the developing child. With respect to

Table 3–3
Activities Hypotheses

Independent Variable	With Friends		Alone	
	Physical	Nonphysical	Physical	Nonphysical
Home Influences				
Parental volunteer work index	+	+	+	+
One-adult household	−	+	0	+
Three or more adults in household	0	0	−	−
Family income over $20,000	+	+	−	−
Family income over $40,000	+	+	−	−
Caregiver has some college	+	−	+	−
Caregiver went to graduate school	+	−	+	−
Caregiver employed outside home	−	0	−	+
Child Factors				
Child's age	−	0	−	0
Child is male	+	−	+	−
Child is White	0	0	0	0
Child is Black	0	0	0	0
Seriousness of illness				
Relatively minor	+	+	+	−
Very severe	−	−	−	+
Number of playmates	+	+	0	−
Environment				
State of Alabama	0	0	0	0

this concept, a multiple-regression analysis found that children who engaged in neighborhood activities with other children had higher self-esteem scores (.723, $p < .01$), enhanced skill development (0.138, $p < .05$), and a sense of support from peers (.328, $p < .01$).

Table 3-4 reports OLS regression analyses explaining each activity scale, physical versus nonphysical, both with friends and alone. Precursor variables better explain activities with friends (38% of the

Table 3–4
Regression Analyses: Activities by Setting

Independent Variable	With Friends		Alone	
	Physical	Nonphysical	Physical	Nonphysical
Intercept	0.668[3]	0.410	0.686[4]	1.575
Home Influences				
Parental Volunteer	−0.003	0.065[1]	−0.025	−0.008
work index	(−0.08)	(1.85)	(−1.08)	(−0.28)
One-adult household	−0.360[1]	0.235	0.010	−0.194
	(−2.03)	(1.52)	(0.10)	(−1.42)
Three or more adults	−0.250	0.134	0.021	−0.332[2]
in household	(−1.42)	(0.87)	(0.20)	(−2.44)
Family income over	−0.115	0.091	−0.066	−0.002
$20,000	(−0.66)	(0.59)	(−0.65)	(−0.01)
Family income over	−0.206	0.259[1]	0.097	−0.116
$40,000	(−1.26)	(1.81)	(1.02)	(−0.92)
Caregiver has some	−0.055	0.017	0.017	0.118
college	(−0.34)	(0.12)	(0.18)	(0.95)
Caregiver went to	0.005	−0.274	−0.047	0.128
graduate school	(0.02)	(−1.61)	(−0.41)	(0.86)
Caregiver employed	−0.028	0.132	−0.204[2]	0.318[2]
outside home	(−0.20)	(1.08)	(−2.50)	(2.96)
Child Factors				
Child over 9 years	−0.136[1]	0.126[3]	−0.092[1]	0.090
of age	(−2.14)	(2.27)	(−2.49)	(1.83)
Child is male	0.635[2]	−0.508[2]	0.215[2]	−0.325[2]
	(4.92)	(−4.50)	(2.85)	(−3.26)
Child is White	0.178	−0.415[3]	0.191	0.152
	(0.76)	(−2.02)	(1.40)	(0.84)
Child is Black	−0.020	−0.595[4]	0.139	0.030
	(−0.08)	(−2.58)	(0.90)	(0.15)
Seriousness of illness				
Relatively minor	0.107	−0.198	−0.014	0.211
	(0.68)	(−1.45)	(−0.15)	(1.74)
Very severe	0.027	−0.157	−0.046	0.177
	(0.18)	(−1.20)	(−0.52)	(1.53)
Number of playmates	0.409[2]	0.243[2]	0.000	0.031
	(11.76)	(7.98)	(0.02)	(1.16)
Environment				
State of Alabama	0.051	0.173	0.009	−0.203
	(0.36)	(1.42)	(0.11)	(−1.89)
R^2 =	.377[4]	.271[4]	.092[3]	.130[4]
R^2 adjusted =	.346	.234	.047	.086
N = 336 df = 16				
Mean =	1.598	0.949	0.565	1.917

[1] Significant at .05 level, one-tailed test of directional hypothesis.
[2] Significant at .01 level, one-tailed test of directional hypothesis.
[3] Significant at .05 level, two-tailed test of null hypothesis.
[4] Significant at .01 level, two-tailed test of null hypothesis.

variance in physical activities, 27% in nonphysical activities) than those done alone (9% in physical, 13% in nonphysical).

Home influences are not strong predictors. Parental volunteer work and family income are shown to only weakly explain passive activities with friends. One-adult households are associated with fewer physical activities with friends; multiple-adult households appear to strongly discourage passive activities alone. Caregiver employment outside the home affects activities alone, encouraging nonphysical but reducing physical activities.

Child factors have more explanatory power. Having more playmates has the strongest associations with both physical and nonphysical activities with friends. Older children clearly engage in fewer physical, but more nonphysical, activities. As expected, the same pattern holds for males. Both White and Black children average fewer nonphysical activities with friends than do children of other racial/ethnic backgrounds.

Table 3-5 gives findings for all activities, alone and with friends. One-adult households are associated with fewer physical activities; multiple-adult household with fewer overall activities. Caregiver employment is associated with fewer nonphysical activities and fewer activities overall. Following the patterns from Table 3-4, older children and females engage in fewer physical but more nonphysical activities. Black children appear to engage in fewer nonphysical activities. Children with more playmates do more activities of all types.

Table 3-6 reports findings for all activities, by level of activity (levels 1 through 4). Not surprisingly, level 1—the most general, lowest-level activities (going outside, role playing)—is not as well explained (6% of variance) as the more specific, higher-level activities (9% to 19%). Of home influences, only being in a one-adult household is associated with physical activities, which are fewer at level 2 (e.g., baseball) and level 3 (e.g., football).

Child factors have greater influence. Older children engage less in general play (level 1 and level 3, and perhaps level 4, e.g., basketball), supporting the idea that the decline in physical activities with age is related to a shift from generalized play to more organized, specialized sports, in which not all children participate with equal ease. Boys participate more than girls in high-level, specific activities

Table 3–5
Regression Analyses: Activities with Friends or Alone

Independent Variable	Activities with Friends or Alone		
	Physical	Nonphysical	Total
Intercept	1.216[4]	2.079[4]	3.295[4]
Home Influences			
Parental volunteer work index	−0.015	0.031	0.016
	(−0.36)	(0.68)	(0.32)
One-adult household	−0.402[1]	0.138	−0.264
	(−2.12)	(0.68)	(−1.20)
Three or more adults in household	−0.273	−0.230	−0.503[3]
	(−1.46)	(−1.15)	(−2.30)
Family income over $20,000	−0.206	0.055	−0.152
	(−1.10)	(0.27)	(−0.69)
Family income over $40,000	−0.135	0.132	−0.003
	(−0.78)	(0.71)	(−0.02)
Caregiver has some college	−0.016	0.120	0.104
	(−0.10)	(0.65)	(0.52)
Caregiver went to graduate school	−0.007	−0.230	−0.224
	(−0.04)	(−1.15)	(−0.93)
Caregiver employed outside home	−0.094	0.440[2]	0.346[1]
	(−0.63)	(2.77)	(1.99)
Child Factors			
Child over 9 years of age	−0.224[2]	0.215[4]	−0.009
	(−3.31)	(2.99)	(−0.11)
Child is male	0.723[2]	−0.802[2]	−0.079
	(5.24)	(−5.46)	(−0.50)
Child is White	0.306	−0.310	−0.004
	(1.22)	(−1.16)	(−0.01)
Child is Black	0.071	−0.600[3]	−0.529
	(0.25)	(−2.00)	(−1.61)
Seriousness of illness			
Relatively minor	0.160	−0.009	0.151
	(0.95)	(−0.05)	(0.77)
Very severe	0.074	−0.031	0.043
	(0.46)	(−0.18)	(0.23)
Number of playmates	0.389[2]	0.231[2]	0.620[2]
	(10.49)	(5.84)	(14.35)
Environment			
State of Alabama	0.001	−0.115	−0.115
	(0.01)	(−0.73)	(−0.66)
R^2 = .351[4]	.241[4]	.418[4]	
R^2 adjusted =	.319	.203	.389
N = 336 df = 16			
Mean =	1.982	2.664	4.646

[1] Significant at .05 level, one-tailed test of directional hypothesis.
[2] Significant at .01 level, one-tailed test of directional hypothesis.
[3] Significant at .05 level, two-tailed test of null hypothesis.
[4] Significant at .01 level, two-tailed test of null hypothesis.

Table 3-6
Regression Analysis: Physical Activities by Level

Independent Variable	Physical Activities by Level			
	Level 1	Level 2	Level 3	Level 4
Intercept	0.561[4]	0.019	0.201	0.436[3]
Home Influences				
Parental volunteer work	−0.015	−0.006	0.004	0.001
index	(−0.69)	(−0.36)	(0.21)	(0.05)
One-adult household	0.002	−0.136[1]	−0.313[2]	0.044
	(0.03)	(−1.81)	(−3.39)	(0.37)
Three or more adults in	0.035	−0.039	−0.127	−0.142
household	(0.37)	(−0.52)	(−1.39)	(−1.22)
Family income over	−0.027	0.037	−0.064	−0.152
$20,000	(−0.29)	(0.49)	(−0.70)	(−1.30)
Family income over	−0.039	−0.043	−0.057	0.003
$40,000	(−0.44)	(−0.62)	(−0.67)	(0.03)
Caregiver has some	0.103	−0.003	−0.006	0.110
college	(1.19)	(−0.05)	(−0.08)	(−1.03)
Caregiver went to	−0.038	0.015	−0.024	0.040
graduate school	(−0.37)	(0.18)	(−0.24)	(0.31)
Caregiver employed	−0.068	−0.080	0.050	0.004
outside home	(−0.91)	(−1.35)	(0.68)	(0.05)
Child Factors				
Child over 9 years	−0.071[1]	0.005	−0.089[2]	−0.068
of age	(−2.11)	(0.18)	(−2.69)	(−1.63)
Child is male	−0.011	0.207[2]	0.321[2]	0.207[2]
	(−0.17)	(3.79)	(4.78)	(2.41)
Child is White	0.040	0.102	0.012	0.152
	(0.32)	(1.03)	(0.10)	(0.98)
Child is Black	−0.213	0.100	0.162	0.021
	(−1.51)	(0.90)	(1.18)	(0.12)
Seriousness of illness:				
Relatively minor	0.081	−0.002	0.073	0.007
	(0.96)	(−0.03)	(0.90)	(0.07)
Very severe	0.046	−0.038	0.161[5]	−0.095
	(0.57)	(−0.60)	(2.07)	(−0.96)
Number of playmates	0.033[1]	0.064[2]	0.098[2]	0.195[2]
	(1.77)	(4.33)	(5.42)	(8.46)
Environment				
State of Alabama	0.103	−0.010	0.000	−0.093
R^2 =	.062	.132[4]	.202[4]	.229[4]
R^2 adjusted =	.015	.089	.162	.191
N = 336 df = 16				
Mean =	0.491	0.289	0.461	0.741

[1] Significant at .05 level, one-tailed test, directional hypothesis.
[2] Significant at .01 level, one-tailed test, directional hypothesis.
[3] Significant at .05 level, two-tailed test, null hypothesis.
[4] Significant at .01 level, two-tailed test, null hypothesis.
[5] Significant at .05 level, two-tailed test, contradicting hypothesis.

(levels 2 to 4); they show essentially no difference in general play. An apparent effect of illness severity is an unexpected higher participation in level 3 activity by the more severely ill. As always, children with more playmates engage in more physical activities at all levels. A stronger relationship exists at higher levels of physical activity.

Many types of activities are not reported at all by considerable proportions of children (see Table 3-2). In such cases, OLS regression results may be biased by censorship at zero—children with no activities may vary in their "distance" from engaging in them, but they cannot have fewer than zero activities. Further, what explains engaging at all may differ from what explains number of activities undertaken. Table 3-7 reports tobit analysis, truncated regression, and probit analysis of numbers of physical activities of all types in which children engage. Tobit analysis adjusts for censorship at zero. Table 3-7 shows some slightly different estimates from those in Table 3-5, but the pattern of findings is the same. Thus, any bias due to censoring at zero does not change the basic findings reported above.

The matter is different when separate truncated regression and probit equations are estimated. When used together, these two techniques shows a significantly better explanation than when using tobit analysis alone. The probit analysis estimates effects on the likelihood of engaging in *any* physical activities; truncated regression estimates the numbers of activities among those who engage in at least one. The negative effect of one-adult households on physical activities is due at least in part to fewer activities among children from such households who are involved in at least some physical activities. By contrast, that older children are involved in fewer physical activities is due in large part to their lower likelihood of engaging in any such activities. A third pattern emerges for males and for children with more playmates: they are both more likely to engage in physical activities and to perform more of them if they do any.

SUMMARY (see Table 3–8)

Chronically ill children engage in many levels of activities, including those requiring exertion. Physical activities tend to be done

Table 3–7
Tobit Analysis, Truncated Regression, and Probit Analysis:
Physical Activities with Friends or Alone

Independent Variable	Tobit Analysis	Truncated Regression	Probit Analysis
Intercept	0.983[3]	1.160[4]	1.052[3]
Home Influences			
Parental volunteer work index	−0.020	−0.020	−0.009
	(−0.40)[1]	(−0.40)	(−0.15)
One-adult household	−0.459[1]	−0.437[1]	−0.295
	(−2.04)	(−1.95)	(−1.12)
Three or more adults in household	−0.309	−0.380	−0.112
	(−1.39)	(−1.72)	(−0.42)
Family income over $20,000	−0.314	−0.061	−0.419
	(−1.42)	(−0.29)	(−1.51)
Family income over $40,000	−0.103	−0.192	0.004
	(−0.50)	(−0.94)	(0.002)
Caregiver has some college	0.004	−0.025	−0.060
	(−0.02)	(−0.13)	(−0.24)
Caregiver went to graduate school	−0.002	−0.136	0.247
	(−0.01)	(−0.56)	(0.80)
Caregiver employed outside home	−0.159	0.069	−0.314
	(−0.90)	(0.40)	(−1.41)
Child Factors			
Child over 9 years of age	−0.288[2]	−0.112	−0.344[2]
	(−3.58)	(−1.40)	(−3.41)
Child is male	0.822[2]	0.773[2]	0.482[2]
	(5.03)	(4.62)	(2.50)
Child is White	0.424	0.338	0.346
	(1.41)	(1.05)	(1.08)
Child is Black	0.099	0.258	−0.047
	(0.29)	(0.73)	(−0.13)
Seriousness of illness			
Relatively minor	−0.002	0.276	−0.240
	(−0.01)	(1.47)	(−1.08)
Very severe	0.177	0.178	0.085
	(0.90)	(0.93)	(0.35)
Number of playmates	0.479[2]	0.287[2]	0.620[2]
	(10.69)	(5.97)	(14.35)
Environment			
State of Alabama	−0.044	0.007	−0.017
	(−0.25)	(0.04)	(−0.08)
df = 16			
Mean =	1.982	2.449	
Log-likelihood =	−534.46	−398.70	−116.40
Chi², use of tobit =	38.72[4]		
Chi² for model =			94.40[2]
N =	336	272	336

[1] Significant at .05 level, one-tailed test of directional hypothesis.
[2] Significant at .01 level, one-tailed test of directional hypothesis.
[3] Significant at .05 level, two-tailed test of null hypothesis.
[4] Significant at .01 level, two-tailed test of null hypothesis.

Table 3–8
Structural Equations: Activities and Playmates

Independent Variable	Number of Activities		Number of Playmates
	Physical	Nonphysical	
Intercept	0.826	3.321[4]	0.650
Endogenous Factors			
Number of physical activities		0.936[1]	0.436[1]
		(−1.72)	(2.15)
Number of playmates	0.779[1]	0.549[1]	
	(1.88)	(1.79)	
Exogenous Factors			
Parental volunteer work index	−0.055	0.020	0.096[1]
	(−0.96)	(0.31)	(1.88)
One-adult household	−0.364[1]	−0.232	0.122
	(−1.89)	(−0.84)	(0.49)
Three or more adults in household	−0.345	−0.478[1]	−0.252
	(−1.65)	(−2.14)	(1.01)
Family income over $20,000	− 0.170	− 0.121	
	(−1.16)	(−0.53)	
Family income over $40,000		−0.106	
		(−0.60)	
Caregiver has some college		0.093	
		0.48	
Caregiver went to graduate school		−0.183	
		(−0.91)	
Caregiver employed outside home	−0.097	0.358[1]	0.029
	(−0.62)	(2.02)	(0.15)
Child Factors			
Child over 9 years of age	−0.308.[2]		−0.280[2]
	(−2.64)		(3.02)
Child is male	0.584[2]	−0.113	
	(2.74)	(−0.20)	
Child is Black	−0.306	−0.499[1]	0.315
	(−1.30)	(−2.283)	(1.46)
Seriousness of illness			
Relatively minor	0.173		−0.202
	(0.99)		(−0.92)
Very severe	0.203		−0.312
	(0.97)		(−1.50)
Environment			
State of Alabama		−0.078	0.144
		(0.39)	(0.86)
N = 336			
3 SLS, R² =	.075[4]	.094[4]	.028
Mean =	1.982	2.664	2.402
df =	11	12	11

[1] Significant at .05 level, one-tailed test of directional hypothesis.
[2] Significant at .01 level, one-tailed test of directional hypothesis.
[3] Significant at .05 level, two-tailed test of null hypothesis.
[4] Significant at .01 level, two-tailed test of null hypothesis.

predominantly with others; nonphysical activities are more often engaged in alone.

A model of parental and child influences on activity is successful, especially at explaining activities done with friends. Adult participation and supervision appear important: children who lie in one-adult households and whose principal caregiver works will engage in fewer physical activities, compared to children in dual-parent families. However, child-specific factors are better predictors than home influences. Having more playmates results in performing more physical activities, both because a child is more likely initially to do the activities and because, once so engaged, the child is likely to participate in more physical activities. Boys engage in more physical activities, especially high-level ones, than girls, again both because they are more likely to perform at least one activity and because those involved are likely to perform a greater variety. Older children take part in fewer physical activities and are less likely to engage in any as they shift from undifferentiated play to more specialized sporting activities.

Findings show transitions from home/parent-centered to peer-centered activity, and from undifferentiated play to organized sport, in chronically ill children aged 9 to 13. Findings also suggest that programs might be adopted to encourage physical activities among girls, among children with fewer playmates, among children whose principal caregiver works outside the home, and among older children who are not generally "selected for the team," whether on the playground or in a more organized venue. Certain chronically ill children—those from one-adult households, those with fewer playmates, and girls—might be targeted to encourage involvement in a wider diversity of physical activities.

DISCUSSION

This study examined chronically ill children's activity patterns in more unstructured situations, and the role of functional requirements or sustenal imperatives in maintaining/supporting activity patterns. All of the subsystems need a certain amount of sustenal imperatives to maintain behavioral system balance. The types and amount of functional requirements/sustenal imperatives needed vary with the child's age and status on the health–illness continuum. The nurse, in order to plan interventions, must understand the role of sustenal imperatives/functional requirements in a chronically ill child's development, be aware of what places a child at risk in terms of a diminished supply of sustenal imperatives/functional requirements, and be able to assess a child's status in terms of what is present and what is needed. In this study, variables, the supply source from which a child draws sustenal imperatives, were identified. These included home influences, child factors, and environment (Table 3-3). This categorization effectively organized the empirical literature, provided a descriptive framework for using the JBS Model, and offered guidance for interventions.

Personal attributes of the child were defined as demographic variables, biomedical status, past and present behaviors, activity history, psychological traits, and states associated with physical activity. Determinants that reside or originate in the individual are important because they can identify personal variables or population segments that may be targets for nursing interventions to increase physical activity, or, conversely, they can describe impediments or people resistive to physical activity interventions. It is important for the nurse, as an external regulator, to know what can be changed for whom, and the personal determinants that may make change difficult.

We found, as have other researchers, that school-age children do not voluntarily participate in a significant amount of regular vigorous physical activity during unstructured or leisure time periods (Sallis, Paterson, McKenzie, & Nadar, 1988; Simons-Morton, Parcel, & O'Hara, 1988). We also found that chronically ill girls spend less time in physical activity than do their male peers. Gender differences in the level of physical activity appear to increase as a function of age. The age and.gender differences in activity level suggest the need to examine further the correlates and courses of interindividual variations in children's activity patterns.

There also seemed to be concomitant associations in the population for low activity, years of parental education, and low income. However, the degree to which they signal causal circumstances or a selection-bias effect remains unclear. Further investigation is warranted if demographics associated with activity are to be interpreted as targets for intervention.

The child's biomedical status is an important factor. There needs to be a match between the demands and challenges of the activity, and the abilities, motivation, and judgment of the child. The motor ability to perform the activity, and, more significantly, the agility, endurance, speed, and strength needed, must match with the child's interests and abilities. At present, little information is available.

PSYCHOSOCIAL

Personality characteristics such as achievement, motivation, stress tolerance, social adequacy, movement satisfaction, self-confidence, and independence may be associated with physical activity but were not examined in this study. Self-esteem was examined and found to be associated with a higher level of physical activity. Involvement with other children was strongly associated with physical activity. Parents also appear to be an influence on physical activity.

ENVIRONMENTAL FACTORS

Many of the potentially enabling, reinforcing, and impeding determinants of physical activity could be environmental. This study investigated only a few of those variables. Access to facilities is certainly an issue, as is a lack of time by both the parents and the child. Climate or region of the country could also be a factor. This study found that children in one-adult households participated in fewer activities.

IMPLICATIONS FOR
NURSING INTERVENTION

The group of chronically ill school-age children studied may not be participating in physical activities to their full potential. The study has identified variables that serve as a source of sustenal imperatives/functional requirements for these children. No one variable or category of variables accounted for most of the variance in the children's activity patterns; rather, the variables appeared to interact. Planning effective interventions is therefore more challenging.

Key areas for nursing interventions would be nurturance and stimulation. Nurturance is defined as supporting the child's adaptive behaviors, and stimulation is used to draw out or develop behaviors that do not exist at the time.

Regarding stimulation, nurses could encourage parents to plan daily exercise periods with their children. Nurses can teach parents how to introduce an inactive child to a physical activity such as walking or bicycling, or a new activity such as bowling. Exercise programs for children have little hope for success unless they are enjoyable. For most inactive children, a session of sweating, panting, and straining will prompt a rapid return to the television set and a bag of corn chips. Thus, teaching parents how to plan an exercise program would be of critical importance.

In facilitating nurturance, the nurse provides conditions that support the progressive growth and development of behaviors. Thus, the nurse teaches the parents that having fun while exercising means not being embarrassed. Any activity that causes a child to fail or look deficient in the presence of peers will be rejected. Exercise programs for children with chronic health problems need to emphasize successes. Individual progress is a strong motivating factor, whether in just sticking with the program or increasing the distance walked per week. Children are more likely to continue exercise if progress is visible and is applauded.

Another approach, combining nurturance and stimulation, is for nurses to use the knowledge base related to exercise to plan an intervention program that combines the learning of fitness principles and an activity program. The children can be given information regarding the cardiorespiratory system and the impact that obesity and exercise have on the system. Discussion can focus on the definition of physical fitness, the components of fitness, the benefits of exercise, and the effort it takes to be physically fit. Special programs can be designed for girls or for children with specific diseases. The children can be taught to interpret their own fitness level and become actively involved in planning their fitness program. "Contracts"—students' written agreements to improve their fitness level in a specified time period—can be developed. Modified contracts can be a family activity in which the nurse helps the child and the family to set realistic goals for participation and improvement. Thus, the children become informed decision makers who can plan and carry out their own activity programs.

SCHOLARS WORKING WITH THE JBS MODEL

Dr. Anayis Derdiarian
Director of Nursing Research
Los Angeles County and
   University of Southern
   California Medical Center
Los Angeles, CA

Dr. Bonnie Holaday
School of Nursing
Wichita State University
Wichita, KS 67260-0041

Dr. Nancy Lovejoy
College of Nursing
Science Center
Harbor Campus
University of Massachusetts,
   Boston
100 Morrissey Boulevard
Boston, MA 02125-3393

Dr. Elizabeth Poster
University of Texas, Arlington
Box 19407
Arlington, TX 76019

Dr. Brooke Randell
School of Nursing
University of Washington
Seattle, WA 98195

Dr. Anne Turner-Henson
School of Nursing
University of Alabama,
   Birmingham
University Station
Birmingham, AL 35294

Dr. Diana Wilkie
Department of Physiological
   Nursing
SM-28
University of Washington
Seattle, WA 98195

REFERENCES

Armstrong, R. W., Rosenbaum, P. L., & King, S. (1992). Self-perceived social functions among disabled children and regular classrooms. *Journal of Developmental and Behavioral Pediatrics, 13,* 11–16.

Auger, J. (1976). *Behavioral systems and nursing.* Englewood Cliffs, NJ: Prentice-Hall.

Bar-Or, O. (1990). Disease-specific benefits of training in the child with chronic disease. What is the evidence? *Pediatric Exercise Sciences, 2,* 384-394.

Bar-Or, O., Inbar, O., & Spira, R. (1976). Physiological effects of a sports rehabilitation program on cerebral palsied and post-poliomyelitic adolescents. *Medical Science & Sports, 8,* 157-161.

Bronfenbrenner, U. (1986). Ecology of the family as a context for human development: Research perspectives. *Developmental Psychology, 22,* 723-742.

Bryant, B. K. (1985). The neighborhood walk: Sources of support in middle childhood. *Monographs of the Society for Research in Child Development, 50*(3), Serial #210.

Burton, C. B., & Krantz, M. (1990). Predicting adjustment in middle childhood from early peer status. *Early Child Development and Care, 60,* 89-100.

Cadman, P., Boyle, M., & Szatmari, P. (1987). Chronic illness disability, and mental health and social well-being: Findings of the Ontario Child Health Study. *Pediatrics, 79,* 805-813.

Cadman, D., Rosenbaum, P., Boyle, M., & Offord, D. R. (1991). Children with chronic illness: Family and parent demographic characteristics and psychosocial adjustment. *Pediatrics, 87,* 884-889.

Campaigne, B., Gilliam, T., & Spencer, R. (1984). Effects of physical activity program on metabolic control and cardiovascular fitness in children with insulin-dependent diabetes mellitus. *Diabetes Care, 7,* 57-62.

Challenor, Y. B. (1989). Exercise and sports for the handicapped child. In D. Nudel (Ed.), *Pediatric sports medicine* (pp. 257-270). New York: PMA Publisher.

Crick, N. R., & Ladd, G. W. (1993). Children's perceptions of their peer experiences: Attributions, loneliness, social anxiety, and social avoidance. *Developmental Psychology, 29,* 244-254.

Dorchy, H., & Poortman, J. (1989). Sport and the diabetic child. *Sports Medicine, 7,* 248-262.

Drake, D. D., & Kuntzleman, C. T. (1988). Early intervention/prevention in childhood. In L. K. Hall & G. C. Meyers (Eds.), *Epidemiology behavior, change, and intervention in chronic disease* (pp. 25-48). Champaign, IL: Life Enhancement.

Fink, G., Kaye, C., Blau, H., & Spitzer, S. A. (1993). Assessment of exercise capacity in asthmatic children with various degrees of activity. *Pediatric Pulmonology, 15,* 41-43.

Garbanino, J. (1985). Habitats for children: An ecological perspective. In J. F. Wohlwill & W. van Vliet (Eds.), *Habitats for children: The impacts of density*. Hillsdale, NJ: Erlbaum.

Gennaro, S., Brooten, D., Klein A., Stringer, M., York, R., & Brown, L. (1993). Cost burden of low birthweight. In S. G. Funk, E. M. Tornquist, M. T. Champagne, R. A. Wieser (Eds.), *Key aspects of caring for the chronically ill* (pp. 271–280). New York: Springer.

Goldberg, B. (1990). Children, sports, and chronic disease. *Physician Sportsmed, 18,* 44–56.

Gortmaker, S. L., Dietz, W. H., & Cheung, L. W. Y. (1990). Inactivity, diet, and the fattening of America. *Journal of the American Dietetic Association, 90,* 1247–1255.

Grubbs, J. (1980). An interpretation of the Johnson Behavioral System Model for nursing practice. In J. Riehl & C. Roy (Eds.), *Conceptual models for nursing practice* (2nd ed., pp. 217–253). New York: Appleton-Century-Crofts.

Hart, R. (1977). *Children's experience of place.* New York: Wiley.

Hobbs, N., Perrin, J., & Ireys, H. T. (1985). *Chronically ill children and their families.* San Francisco: Jossey-Bass.

Hochschild, A. (1989). *The second shift.* New York: Viking Press.

Holaday, B., & Turner-Henson, A. (1989). Response effects in surveys with school-age children. *Nursing Research, 38,* 248–250.

Holaday, B., Turner-Henson, A., & Swan, J. (1991). Stability of school-age children's survey responses. *Image: The Journal of Nursing Scholarship, 23,* 109–114.

Jessop, D. J., Riesmann, C. K., & Stein, R. E. K. (1988). Chronic childhood illness and maternal mental health. *Journal of Developmental and Behavioral Pediatrics, 9,* 147–156.

Johnson, D. E. (1980). The behavioral system model for nursing. In J. Riehl & C. Roy (Eds.), *Conceptual model for nursing practice* (2nd ed., pp. 207–216). New York: Appleton-Century-Crofts.

Johnson, D. E. (1990). The behavioral system model for nursing. In M. Parker (Ed.), *Nursing theories in practice* (pp. 23–32). New York: National League for Nursing Press.

Landau, S., & Milich, R. (1990). Assessment of children's social status and peer relations. In A. M. LaGreca (Ed.), *Through the eyes of the child: Obtaining self-reports from children and adolescents* (pp. 259–291). Needham Heights, MA: Allyn & Bacon.

Larigne, J. V., & Faier-Routman, J. (1992). Psychological adjustment to pediatric physical disorders: A meta-analytic review. *Journal of Pediatric Psychology, 17,* 133–157.

Lennard, H. L., & Lennard, S. H. (1992). Children in public places: Some lessons from European cities. *Children's Environments, 9*(2), 37-39.

Marcenko, M. O., & Meyers, J. C. (1991). Mothers of children with developmental disabilities: Who shares the burden? *Family Relations, 40,* 186-190.

Mayo, L. (1956). *Problem and challenge: Guides to action on chronic illness.* New York: National Health.

Medrich, E., Roizen, J., Rubin, V., & Buckley, S. (1982). *The serious business of growing up: A study of children's lives outside of school.* Berkeley: University of California Press.

Moore, L. L., Lombardi, M. J., White, M. J., Campbell, J. L., Oliveria, S. A., & Ellison, R. C. (1991). Influence of parents' physical activity levels on activity levels of young children. *Journal of Pediatrics, 118,* 215-219.

Noll, R. B., Rio, M. D., Daives, W. H., Bukowski, W. M., & Koontz, K. (1992). Social interactions between children with cancer or sickle cell disease and their peers: Teacher ratings. *Journal of Developmental and Behavioral Pediatrics, 13,* 187-193.

Noschis, K. (1992). Child development theory and planning for neighborhood play. *Children's Environments, 9*(2), 3-9.

Orenstein, D. M., Reed, M. E., Grogan, F. T., Jr., & Crawford, L. V. (1985). Exercise conditioning in children with asthma. *Journal of Pediatrics, 106,* 556-560.

Paterson, M. A. (1993). The financial impact of disability on the family: Issues and interventions. *Family & Community Health, 16,* 46-55.

Pless, I. B., Power, C., & Peckham, C. S. (1993). Long-term psychosocial sequelae of chronic physical disorders in childhood. *Pediatrics, 91,* 1131-1136.

Ross, J. G., & Pate, R. (1987). The national children and youth fitness study: A summary of the findings. *Journal of Physical Education, Recreation and Dance, 56,* 51-56.

Rutenfranz, J., Anderson, K. L., Seliger, V., & Masironi, R. (1982). Health standards in terms of exercise fitness of school children in urban and rural areas in various European countries. *Annals of Clinical Research, 34,* 33-36.

Sallis, J., Simons-Morton, B., Stone, E., Corbin, C., (1992). Determinants of physical activity and interventions in youth. *Medicine and Science in Sports and Exercise, 24,* 524-525.

Sallis, J. F., Patterson, T. L., McKenzie, T. L., & Nader, P. R. (1988). Family variables and physical activity in preschool children. *Journal of Developmental and Behavioral Pediatrics, 9,* 57-61.

Simons-Morton, B., Parcel, G., & O'Hara, N. (1988). Health-related physical fitness in childhood: Status and recommendations. *Annual Review of Public Health, 9,* 403–425.

Stein, R., & Jessop, D. J. (1989). What a diagnosis does not tell: The case for a noncategorical approach to chronic illness in childhood. *Social Science Medicine, 29,* 769–778.

Stevens, M. S. (1994). Parents coping with infants requiring home cardiorespiratory monitoring. *Journal of Pediatric Nursing, 9,* 2–12.

Streitmatter, J. L., & Pate, G. S. (1989). Identity status development and cognitive prejudice in early adolescents. *Journal of Early Adolescence, 9,* 142–152.

Turner-Henson, A., Holaday, B., & O'Sullivan, P. (1992). Sampling rare pediatric populations. *Journal of Pediatric Nursing, 7,* 329–334.

Turner-Henson, A., Holaday, B., & Swan, J. (1992). When parenting becomes caregiving: Caring for the chronically ill child. *Family & Community Health, 15,* 19–30.

Updyke, W., & Willett, M. (1989). *Physical fitness trends in American youth, 1989-1990.* Bloomington, IN: Chrysler–AAU Physical Fitness Program. (Press Release)

U.S. Bureau of the Census (1995a). *Household and family characteristics: March 1994* (Current Population Reports Series P-20, No. 437). Washington, DC: U.S. Government Printing Office.

U.S. Bureau of the Census (1995b). *Marital status and living arrangements: March 1994* (Current Population Reports Series P-20, No. 433). Washington, DC: U.S. Government Printing Office.

U.S. Department of Labor (1994). *Facts on women workers.* Washington, DC: U.S. Government Printing Office.

Weiland, S. K., Pless, I. B., & Roughman, K. J. (1992). Chronic illness and mental health problems in pediatric practice. *Pediatrics, 89,* 445–450.

Weinstein, C., & David, T. G. (1986). *Spaces for children: The built environment and child development.* New York: Plenum.

Woods, N. F., Yates, B. C., & Primono, J. (1984). Supporting families during chronic illness. *Image: The Journal of Nursing Scholarship, 21,* 46–50.

4

The Roy Adaptation Model in Research: Rehabilitation Nursing

Stacey Hoffman Barone and Callista Roy

*T*he Roy Adaptation Model is a nursing theoretical framework that provides a solid foundation for scholarly knowledge development in nursing, the conduct of research, and the guidance of nursing practice as a scientific discipline. Utilization of the model as a theoretical framework fosters organized, comprehensive research in further understanding the basic life processes that promote health and healing or the basic science of nursing. The model also promotes an understanding of the process of coping during health and illness, and the enhancement of adaptive coping or the clinical science of nursing. This chapter presents a blueprint of model-based research. The exemplar used to demonstrate the implementation of the blueprint is a research study in rehabilitation nursing (Barone, 1993), which utilized the Roy Adaptation Model as its theoretical framework. Through the use of this example, the authors will discuss the process of model application to research and the critical factors to consider when selecting, applying, and evaluating a theoretical framework to guide research for nursing.

The utilization of a nursing theoretical framework to conduct research encourages the investigator to look beyond the boundaries of the research and contemplate the interaction of the person, environment, nursing, and health as represented in the model itself. This is critical for sound, thorough research in nursing. Nursing is a relatively young scientific discipline; accordingly, research activities are often conducted by novice researchers. A nursing theoretical framework provides a new researcher with a reference point for the concepts that will be studied, their interrelationships, and the key questions for inquiry. It encourages critical inquiry, conceptual clarity, and comprehensive visions about the phenomena of concern to the discipline of nursing.

A complete understanding of the components of the model and its functioning as an entity is necessary for its use as a theoretical framework for nursing research. The philosophical and scientific underpinnings of the nursing model should be congruent with the foundational concepts of the specialty of nursing in which the research is being conducted. The researcher must be comfortable with the definitions and relationships of person, environment, nursing, and health and healing as presented within the model, and the application thereof to the research.

Rehabilitation nursing adopts a holistic definition of nursing, viewing the person as a biopsychosocial spiritual and behavioral being. The Association of Rehabilitation Nurses defines their practice as facilitating individuals, through optimum adaptation, to reengage themselves in the mainstream of living whereby the client functions maximally within his or her environment. Dittmar (1989) defines the goal of rehabilitation nursing as facilitating the movement of individuals toward independence while helping them satisfy their needs. The Roy Adaptation Model views the person as a holistic, adaptive system, while also representing the person as a biobehavioral and spiritual being. As the philosophical components of the Roy Adaptation Model are explored herein, the philosophical fit of the Roy Adaptation Model and rehabilitation nursing will become apparent.

OVERVIEW OF THE ROY ADAPTATION MODEL

The philosophic assumptions of the Roy Adaptation Model are based on the principles of humanism and veritivity. The scientific assumptions are predicated on von Bertalanffy's (1968) general systems theory and on Helson's (1964) adaptation level theory.

Humanism is defined by Roy (1988) as the broad movement in philosophy and psychology that recognizes the person and subjective dimensions of the human experience as central to knowing and valuing, and serves as the basis for the following four specific assumptions. In humanism, it is believed that the individual (a) shares in creative power; (b) behaves purposefully, not in a sequence of cause and effect; (c) possesses intrinsic holism; and (d) strives to maintain integrity and to realize the need for relationships (Roy, 1988).

The concept of veritivity is defined by Roy (1988) as a principle of human nature that affirms a common purposefulness of human existence. In veritivity, it is believed that the individual in society is viewed in the context of (a) the purposefulness of human existence, (b) the unity of purpose of humankind, (c) the activity and creativity for the common good, and (d) the value and meaning of life. A belief in something absolute outside oneself allows one to reach to the infinite rather than posing limits to the possibilities of human nature.

Fundamental components of systems theory, such as inputs, outputs, control, and feedback processes, contribute to the Roy Adaptation Model. The person is an adaptive system functioning with interdependent parts that work together for a unified purpose. Adaptation-level theory provides the basis for understanding that the individual as a system has the capacity to adapt to and change or affect the environment (Roy & Andrews, 1991). The ability to respond positively to changes in a function of the person's adaptation level, which is a changing point influenced by the demands of the situation and the person's internal resources, including capabilities, hopes, dreams, aspirations, motivations, and all that makes the person constantly move toward mastery (Roy, 1990).

Combining systems theory and adaptation theory with respect to the concept of the person allows nursing to view the individual as a holistic adaptive system. Holism refers to the idea that the human system is functioning as a whole, despite its interdependent parts. Roy refers to inputs for the person as stimuli that may come externally from the environment or internally from the self. The pooling of stimuli creates a specific input, which is termed the person's adaptation level. The output is a response to the pooled incoming stimuli processed through the person's adaptation level. The primary mechanisms for processing stimuli, both internal and external, are the regulator and the cognator mechanisms (Roy & Andrews, 1991). The person's behavior is presented as adaptive or ineffective responses and results from cognator and regulator processing.

Roy refers to the environment as the world surrounding and within the person. Environment is further broken down into three types of stimuli: (a) focal, (b) contextual, and (c) residual. The focal stimulus is the internal or external stimulus most immediately confronting the person (Roy & Andrews, 1991). For example, the focal stimulus of pain for the oncology rehabilitation patient must be managed effectively to permit participation in therapy. Essentially, the focal stimulus of pain must be replaced by the focal stimulus of therapy.

Contextual stimuli are all other stimuli present in the situation; however, these stimuli are not the focus of the person's attention or energy. Contextual stimuli influence the person's coping responses to the focal stimulus and can present as positive or negative influences. For example, hunger or a loud therapy environment as contextual stimuli may distract the rehabilitation patient from concentrating on therapy.

Residual stimuli are environmental factors within or outside the person, the effects of which, in the current situation, are not determined. Recalling a relative's difficult experience with cancer may stimulate anxiety in the patient without the patient's making the association between current feelings and the past situation. Likewise, the health care provider may not recognize the cues of anxiety and consequently not provide the individual with the opportunity to explore past experiences. Residual stimuli may include the nurse's intuitive impressions regarding the patient's behavioral influences.

The three types of stimuli—focal, contextual, and residual—combine to create the person's adaptation level. The person's response to any situation, such as illness or injury, depends on these three types of stimuli and their current influence on the person. These stimuli determine a range of coping for the person. Coping mechanisms are defined as both innate and acquired ways of responding to the changing environment. Innate coping mechanisms are genetically determined or common to the species, and are generally viewed as automatic processes; the person does not have to think about them. Perspiring on a hot day is the body's way of cooling down, yet the person does not have to consciously request the body to perspire. Acquired coping mechanisms are developed through processes such as learning, in which life experiences contribute to customary responses to particular stimuli. Acquired coping results in deliberate, conscious responses. The warm patient removes his or her sweatshirt to cool down. This action is an acquired coping response.

Innate and acquired coping mechanisms are grouped into two subsystems, the regulator and the cognator (Roy & Andrews, 1991). The regulator subsystem responds automatically through neural, chemical, and endocrine coping processes. Internal and external environmental stimuli perceived through the senses function as inputs to the nervous system. These inputs affect the fluid and electrolyte and endocrine systems, creating automatic, unconscious responses. Concurrently, the regulator subsystem receives input to form perceptions.

A patient who has sustained a spinal cord injury that has resulted in paralysis may feel anxiety when he hears an unexpected individual enter his room at night. His pupils will dilate to enhance his vision, and his heart rate will accelerate as a stress response, making him more alert. This regulator system activity facilitates self-protection by enhancing the senses and preparing the individual for potential self-defense activity if necessary.

The cognator subsystem receives input from both the internal and external stimuli. The stimuli involve psychological, social, physical, and physiological factors, and they initiate four kinds of cognitive-emotive channels: (a) perceptual/information processing, (b) learning, (c) judgment, and (d) emotion. Initially, the cognator interacts with perceptual inputs of the regulator. Perceptual/information processing continues through such activities as selective attention, coding, and memory. Learning involves imitation, reinforcement, and insight; judgment encompasses activities such as problem solving and decision making. The person's emotional response is composed of defenses that are used to reduce anxiety and develop affective appraisal and attachments.

The responses to environmental stimuli are termed behavior and are defined as internal or external actions and reactions under specified circumstances. Output behavior exemplifies the quality of adaptation to environmental change. Adaptive responses are those that promote the integrity of the person in terms of the goals of adaptation: survival, growth, reproduction, and mastery. Ineffective responses are those that do not promote the integrity of the person nor contribute to the goals of adaptation (Roy & Andrews, 1991). Nursing interacts with the person as a holistic adaptive system. Roy describes adaptation as a process designed to foster positive health effects through holistic functioning. The person has four modes of adaptation: (a) physiologic needs, (b) self-concept, (c) role function, and (d) interdependence. Roy (Riehl & Roy, 1980) defines a mode as a method of doing or acting; thus, a mode of adaptation is a way of adapting.

The physiological mode is associated with the way the person responds physically to stimuli from the environment. Behavior in this mode is the manifestation of the physiological activity of all the cells, tissues, organs, and systems comprising the human body (Roy & Andrews, 1991). Roy describes five needs related to physiological integrity: (a) oxygenation, (b) nutrition, (c) elimination, (d) activity, and (e) rest and protection. Also inherent in a discussion of physiological adaptation are complex regulating processes involving senses, fluids and electrolytes, and neurological and endocrine function.

A patient with a spinal cord injury provides an example of changes in the physiological mode, particularly in loss of motor and sensory functioning. Roy and Andrews (1991) define activity as body movement that serves various purposes, such as carrying out daily living chores and protecting self or others from bodily injuries. Activity involves the structures of normal movement: the voluntary and autonomic neuromuscular and skeletal systems. Activity also involves the motivation to move and a free nonrestrictive environment in which to move. Physical activity contributes to the maintenance of all the major body functions. It promotes the normal oxygenation process by stimulating cardiovascular circulation and proper lung expansion with mobilization of its secretions. It maintains the muscle tone of the musculoskeletal system, promotes normal flow through the urinary tract, stimulates the gastric mobility needed for proper digestion and elimination, and facilitates the maintenance of a normal metabolic rate.

The self-concept mode, one of three psychosocial modes, focuses specifically on the psychological and spiritual aspects of the person. The basic need underlying the self-concept mode is psychic integrity, or the need to know one's identity so that one can be or exist with a sense of unity. Self-concept is defined as the composite beliefs and feelings that one holds about oneself at a given time. Formed from perceptions, particularly of the reactions of others, self-concept directs the person's behavior (Driever, 1976). Self-concept is the mediator between the external and internal worlds of the person. Self-concept has two components: (a) the physical self, which includes body sensations and body image, and (b) the personal self, which includes self-consistency, self-ideal/self-expectancy, and moral-ethical-spiritual self. The individual who has sustained a spinal cord injury with paralysis experiences a psychological adjustment to the body changes that have occurred, such as restricted motor function and sensory impairment. The adjustment impacts on the physical self of one's self-concept. Equally important is the introspection that often occurs after a catastrophic illness, resulting in a revisiting of one's purpose, responses, capabilities, beliefs, and sense of self, thus affecting the personal self of one's self-concept.

Role function is the performance of duties based on given positions within society. The way one performs these duties is constantly responsive to external interaction. Each role exists in relationship to another. The basic need underlying the role function mode has been identified as social integrity or the need to know who one is in relation to others so that one can act. The physical restrictions often imposed by a spinal cord injury can create barriers to current vocations. For example, a self-employed plumber who supported his family and ran his own business independently was forced to evaluate new career options after sustaining a spinal cord injury. He eventually pursued computer science as a vocation.

Finally, in relation to others, the person adapts according to a system of interdependence. This system involves ways of seeking help, attention, affection, affirmation, belonging, approval, and understanding. It focuses on interactions related to the giving and receiving of love, respect, and value. Roy and Andrews (1991) describe the basic need of this mode as *affectional adequacy* or a feeling of security in nurturing relationships. Two specific relationships are the focus of the interdependence mode: (a) significant others and (b) support systems. The catastrophic nature of a spinal cord injury subjects the patient to complex changes in personhood. These adjustments include how he or she relates to others with a new sense of self. Relating to others, interacting, and being loved are all part of the social world of individuals. Changes in one's most intimate relationships—with significant others, parents, children, and friends—occur with the change in self in response to illness. These changes can represent opportunities for growth and development in the areas of relating, loving, and belonging. Interaction with one's world is now experienced through the lens of the new experience, and the relating that occurs is the focus of the interdependence mode.

THE ROY MODEL AS A BASIS FOR RESEARCH

The purpose of nursing research is to develop knowledge for nursing practice. The Roy Adaptation Model contributes to nursing as a scholarly practice discipline by guiding research in understanding the basic life processes that promote health—that is, the basic science of nursing—and in discovering how persons cope with health and illness and what can be done to enhance adaptive coping—that is, the clinical science of nursing. The general perspective on nursing knowledge described by Roy (1988) involves focusing on human

life processes from which life patterns emerge and emphasizing related clinical theories, including middle-range theories, of intervention and approaches to enhancing positive life processes and
patterns.

According to the Roy Adaptation Model, basic nursing knowledge
is understanding people who are adapting within their various life
situations. Adaptation is a function of the processes of the cognator
and regulator subsystems and is manifested in the four adaptive
modes. Thus, basic nursing science derived from the model seeks to
describe, explain, and predict how persons function as adaptive systems and exhibit their levels of adaptation. Understanding cognator
and regulator activity, and behaviors and stimuli in each of the adaptive modes, is basic knowledge within the model. The clinical science extends this understanding to particular clinical populations
facing the challenges of their health conditions. The nurse investigator seeks to understand human processes in given health situations, and to build and test theories of how nurses can help persons,
families, and groups enhance their adaptation.

In addition to defining the content of nursing research, the Roy
Adaptation Model is useful in providing a prospective for research
strategies. Nurse researchers use both qualitative and quantitative
designs in their studies. They recognize that these two approaches
are complementary. Qualitative designs see reality as emerging and
as interpretive. The Roy model assumes a focus on individual experiences and the understanding of the context for the person in any
adaptive situation. Qualitative designs are not only consistent with
the model but are often required to answer significant research
questions generated by the model. For example, the model has identified self-consistency as an important component of the self-
concept mode. Some theoretical work has described the broad
characteristics of self-consistency. However, much research is
needed to describe self-consistency in different populations, to relate self-consistency to changes in health status, and to delineate
nursing approaches to dealing with individuals to strengthen self-
consistency as a reflection of an adaptive pattern. If the investigator
wants to describe self-consistency of the adolescent, a qualitative
methodology is warranted to uncover the specific themes related to
self-consistency in this age group. Roy used qualitative methods in

her own work. For example, content analysis of field observations and interview of mothers with their children in the playroom of a hospital was used to describe and define the concept of role adequacy. This concept was later used as a basis for tool development in a quantitative study of the changes in the level of role adequacy of mothers of hospitalized children (Roy, 1967).

Quantitative research designs see reality as discovered and verified. The Roy Adaptation Model assumes that the adaptive processes and patterns of the individual can be recognized in human behavior that is open to observation. Furthermore, the model presupposes a belief in commonalities of patterns of person–environment interactions. Observation and generalizations are basic to quantitative research methods. Thus, quantitative research designs are useful in developing knowledge based on the Roy Adaptation Model. More specifically, the model proposes propositions, that is, relationships between concepts that can be examined by quantitative methods. For example, the model provides the general proposition that the characteristics of the stimuli affect the regulator and cognator coping strategies. In a quantitative research study with low-birth-weight infants, Norris, Campbell, and Brenhert (1982) reported that the nurses' actions of suctioning and positioning have a greater effect on oxygenation need than do other procedures.

Conceptual models that are used in nursing research are particularly significant for the interpretation phase of the research process. Isolated facts, even if they are supported by the canons of good qualitative and quantitative research, do not of themselves provide knowledge. Understanding of the fact is provided by the investigators' interpretation of the facts that have emerged or been discovered. Interpretation is never done in a vacuum. Beliefs about the nature of knowledge, about people and their world, and about the nature of nursing enter into the interpretation of research data. If a conceptual model of nursing has guided the selection of the research question, the variables, and the method of study, then the investigator has a framework for interpreting the results. The data of the research findings can enter the real world of nursing practice by being put into the language of nursing. The conceptual model provides that language. In the suggested study of self-consistency of adolescents, the research could report in a box the themes identified in the

qualitative data collection. However, the meaning of the data becomes clear when the themes are discussed as patterns of self-
consistency in the adolescents' adapting self-concept. Further,
understanding is increased by referring back to the supposition of
the model that these patterns emerge from the thinking and feeling
processes of the cognator, and that they can be influenced by
human experience. Similarly, Norris et al. (1982) present three
graphs of mean TcpO^2. The graphs take on meaning when they are
interpreted as changing oxygenation needs in infants during a time
interval of presentation of three different stimuli. Issues for practice can be raised within this understanding.

The research application that follows provides further illustration
of the use of the Roy Adaptation Model in nursing research. Further,
this example serves as a blueprint for the use of this particular
model in nursing research.

RESEARCH APPLICATION OF THE
ROY ADAPTATION MODEL:
ADAPTATION TO SPINAL CORD INJURY

Selection of a problem to study is one of the most challenging and
crucial tasks faced by the researcher. Fuller (1982) states that good
clinical studies include: frequent and evident occurrence of the
problem in a distinct patient population; a feeling that the current
way of dealing with the problem is unsatisfactory; and a way of reli-
ably measuring any aspect of the problem. In addition, Mateo and
Kirchhoff (1991) suggest evaluating: whether patient care will be
improved as a result of the study; whether adequate human, financial, and environmental resources are available to conduct the
study; and whether the problem is an ethical one.

Clinical experience often is the best source of problem identification for research. In this example, the researcher observed that
the outcome of individuals with spinal cord injuries was not consistently determined by predictive factors identified in the literature,
such as socioeconomic status and education. The researcher repeatedly witnessed individuals utilizing constructive coping mechanisms and adapting well to their spinal cord injury despite a lack of

financial or educational resources, while educated, financially established individuals often participated in self-defeating behaviors. This process of inquiry led to an integrated review of research literature, which stimulated the development of the rationale and research question for this specific research project.

RATIONALE AND PURPOSE OF RESEARCH

Permanent physical disability has long-term consequences that affect the overall well-being of a person. Sustaining a spinal cord injury causes severe disruption of all aspects of an individual's life, resulting in drastic physical limitations and psychosocial isolation. The complex structure of the central nervous system has a limited ability to regenerate. Individuals who sustain damage to their spinal cord face the difficult process of coping with the overwhelming and far-reaching effects of the impairment in order to lead a meaningful life. Research has been conducted to identify the factors that promote physiological and psychological adaptation within various chronically ill populations. Results support a correlation between effective adaptation and the presence of the hardiness personality characteristic (Contrada, 1985; Lee, 1983; Pollock, 1986, 1989b; Pollock & Duffy, 1990). Research also suggests a relationship between an individual's coping abilities and adaptation to stressful events (Boyle, Grap, Younger, & Thornby, 1991; Dew, Lynch, Ernst, Rosenthal, & Judd, 1985; Folkman & Lazarus, 1980, 1985). No similar research has been conducted evaluating hardiness and coping within the spinal cord injured population. The purpose of the research study was to determine the extent to which sociodemographic characteristics and hardiness explain coping, and the extent to which significant predictors of coping explain physiologic and psychosocial adaptation in the individual with a spinal cord injury. The specific aims of the research study were:

1. To determine the extent to which the contextual stimuli of sociodemographic characteristics and the residual stimulus of hardiness explain cognator coping processes in a sample of individuals with spinal cord injuries.

2. To determine the extent to which the significant contextual and residual stimuli that explain coping and the significant cognator coping processes explain physiologic adaptation in a sample of individuals with spinal cord injuries.

3. To determine the extent to which the significant contextual and residual stimuli that explain coping and the significant cognator coping processes explain psychosocial adaptation in a sample of individuals with spinal cord injuries.

Lindeman and Schantz (1982) outline three criteria as being critical in the evaluation of a good research question:

1. The question can be answered by collecting observable data.
2. The question includes the relationship between two or more variables.
3. The question is logical and consistent with what is already known about the subject.

The development of the research question upon completion of a literature review will enlighten the researcher to the significance of and rationale for the study. Identifying and defining the variables within the study are important steps in its empirical design. The variables must be operationalized to ensure their measurement. The Roy Adaptation Model assisted in the process of variable identification and operationalization while providing a structure for understanding the relationship of these variables.

DESIGN OF THE STUDY

A descriptive explanatory design was utilized, consisting of a mailed survey and interview format. Instruments were administered nationally to members of the National Spinal Cord Injury Association. A nonprobability purposive sample, composed of 243 adults, 18 years of age or older, with quadriplegia or paraplegia and a minimum of 4 weeks postinjury, was included.

Figure 4-1 represents the application of the environmental components of the Roy Adaptation Model to the current study. The focal

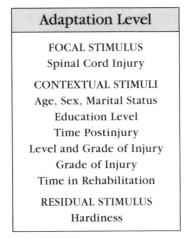

Figure 4–1. The Combined Effects of the Stimuli Create the Adaptation Level of the Individual.

stimulus is the sustained spinal cord injury as experienced by the individual. Although the mean time postinjury for this study's sample was almost 13 years, the widespread and permanent effects of a spinal cord injury impact directly on most aspects of the individual's world, affecting every immediate situation, thereby maintaining its impact as a focal stimulus. Contextual stimuli are those intervening variables, as supported by the literature, that indicate the following relevant demographic data: age, sex, marital status, education level, time postinjury, level and grade (severity) of injury, and time spent in rehabilitation. The residual stimulus selected for evaluation within this study is the hardiness personality characteristic (Kobasa, 1979). This multidimensional construct is represented by the interrelated components of the concepts labeled control, challenge, and commitment. The residual stimulus can be evaluated to determine what internal factors affect the stress response and promote adaptation.

Measurement of the cognator subsystem was undertaken to examine the processes of cognator coping as explained by the effects of the designated focal, contextual, and residual stimuli. In addition, significant predictor stimuli and cognator coping were evaluated to measure what extent of physiologic and psychosocial adaptation could be explained. The concept of the cognator (cognitive/emotive) coping has been operationalized by Folkman and Lazarus (1988) through the Revised Ways of Coping Checklist. The eight mechanisms of coping as described by Folkman and Lazarus are: (a) confrontive, (b) distancing, (c) self-controlling, (d) social support, (e) acceptance of responsibility, (f) escape–avoidance, (g) planful problem solving, and (h) positive reappraisal. Roy has developed a cognator strategies questionnaire (Cognitive Adaptation Processing Scale) and is currently testing it for reliability and validity. At the time of the study, however, the concept of the cognator coping had not been operationalized to the degree of the Lazarus and Folkman tool, hence the use of the Ways of Coping Checklist.

The regulator subsystem participates in the process of creating and influencing perceptions and coping processes. This component of the Roy Adaptation Model, although acknowledged as a vital piece of the system, did not require measurement to meet the aims of the study. Therefore, it was not evaluated.

The outcomes of the individual coping processes were divided between physiologic and psychosocial adaptation. Roy and Andrews (1991) refer to two major categories of assessment factors for the activity portion of the physiologic mode: (a) the type and amount of physical activity carried out by the person and (b) the person's motor function status, which depends on muscle and joint mobility, posture, gait, and coordination. The activity level of the individual was assessed using the modified version of the FONE Functional Independence Measure (Smith, Hamilton, & Granger, 1990). Measurement of physical health in terms of functioning only partially represents physiologic adaptation (Roy & Andrews, 1991). Therefore, measurement of medical complications developed as a result of the management of the condition that affects the physiologic areas—described by Roy as oxygenation, nutrition, elimination, activity, and rest and protection—were included as a partial measurement of physiologic adaptation. Medical complications were assessed using a modified versions of Cyr's (1989) Sequelae of Spinal Cord Injury Instrument. Outcome data from these two components represented physiologic adaptation.

Psychosocial adaptation theoretically includes the three psychosocial modes of the individual: (a) self-concept, (b) role function, and (c) interdependence. The Psychosocial Adjustment to Illness Survey, Self-Report (PAIS-SR) (Derogatis, 1990) assesses seven domains closely aligned with the content of the psychosocial modes of the individual and was developed for utilization with patients who are adapting to illness. It was utilized to measure psychosocial adaptation.

Roy and Andrews (1991) identified a typology of indicators of adaptation for each mode within the model. The researchers compared the indicators from the psychosocial modes with Derogatis's domains and theoretically paired each domain with the content from the indicated mode. The self-concept mode was measured using the PAIS-SR domains of health care orientation, sexual relationships, and psychological distress; the role function mode was measured using the PAIS-SR domains of domestic and vocational environment; and the interdependence mode was measured using the PAIS-SR social environment and family relationships domains. Figure 4–2 is a schematic representation of the application of the

Stimuli	Coping Mechanisms	Responses
FOCAL	COGNATOR	PHYSIOLOGIC
Spinal cord injury	Way of Coping	ADAPTATION
CONTEXTUAL	Checklist:	Fone FIM
Age, sex, marital	Distancing	Functional ability
status	Self-controlling	Medical sequelae
Education level	Social support	Medical complication
Time postinjury	Accepting	PSYCHOSOCIAL
Level and grade of	responsibility	ADAPTATION
injury	Escape–Avoidance	PAIS:
Time in rehabilitation	Planful problem solving	Health care orientation
RESIDUAL	Positive reappraisal	Vocational environment
Hardiness	Confrontive	Domestic environment
Control	REGULATOR	Sexual relationship
Commitment		Family relationship
Challenge		Social environment
		Psychosocial distress

Figure 4–2. Representation and Application of the Components of the Roy Adaptation Model to the Conceptual Variables and Empirical Indicators for Research.

components of the Roy Adaptation Model with the conceptual variables and empirical indicators for research.

FINDINGS

The findings of this study support the use of the Roy Adaptation Model as a conceptual framework to study adaptation to illness in this sample. Exploring the input of adaptive systems in light of the focal stimulus and adaptation level is essential for nursing knowledge development (Roy, 1987). Andrews and Roy's (1986) premise that a person's ability to respond positively or negatively to any given situation depends on the situation, the person's adaptation level, and the individual's coping process, was demonstrated by the study's results.

Study Aim I explored the relationship between two key concepts within the model: the stimuli and the cognator coping processes. Study Aims II and III explored the relationships among three key concepts within the model: (a) the stimuli, (b) the cognator coping processes, and (c) the adaptation outcomes. The following results support the proposed direction of the relationship among the focal, contextual, and residual stimuli (which comprise the adaptation level), the cognator coping mechanisms, and the adaptation outcomes within the Roy Adaptation Model.

The canonical variate results addressing Study Aim I identified a group of subjects with less education and with more recent injuries, who were less hardy in all three dimensions, were more likely to use escape–avoidance coping strategies, and were less likely to seek social support, planful problem solving, and positive reappraisal coping behaviors. The second canonical variate addressing Study Aim I identified a group of younger never-married male subjects who used the confrontive, self-controlling, accepting responsibility, and planful problem solving coping behaviors. The results of Study Aim II identified subjects who had a lower level of spinal cord injury, spent less time in rehabilitation, had a greater sense of control and a higher functional independence score, and experienced less frequent complications. The results of Study Aim III identified younger subjects who had a perceived sense of control; used decreased escape–avoidance, confrontive, and self-controlling coping behaviors; had increased positive reappraisal strategies; and had a greater overall psychosocial adaptation.

PRACTICAL ASPECTS OF THE ROY ADAPTATION MODEL AND ITS FIT WITHIN NURSING RESEARCH AND PRACTICE

The Roy Adaptation Model identifies persons, as individuals and groups, as the phenomena for study. The Roy model and its philosophical assumptions identify a broad perspective of person, including individual holism, interpersonal processes, and the unity of purpose of human life within society. Although nurses typically care for individuals, the principles of the Roy Adaptation Model can be applied to groups, families, communities, and society (Andrews & Roy, 1991). The Roy Adaptation Model has a breadth, scope, and flexibility to be useful across patient populations and to be applied to a wide range of nursing practice settings, from the emergency room to community-based nursing practice. This flexibility is evident from the large number and broad range of research reports currently available in the literature, and from applications to clinical practice in which the Roy Adaptation Model is utilized as a theoretical framework. Although the Roy Adaptation Model is complex, it provides a viewpoint for the research. The elements and assumptions of the Roy Adaptation Model facilitate the choice of phenomena to study and the research questions to be asked. Therefore, the particular setting or specialty of nursing practice should not determine the applicability of the utilization of the model for the research study; rather, the philosophical and conceptual congruence of the model to the practice environment and the chosen patient population should be the determining factor.

One of the challenges that remains in the application of grand nursing theory to nursing research is the empirical measurement of the concepts found within the model. Within this particular study, it was necessary to measure a multitude of concepts and constructs: hardiness, cognator coping, and physiological and psychosocial adaptation. The standardized instruments available for measurement of the concepts and constructs as operationalized in the study were evaluated for content validity. The selected instruments were critiqued for validity and reliability.

Accessibility of instruments for evaluation is a current problem. Although a limited number of books summarize research instruments, locating these resources and subsequently accessing the instruments are often plagued with many barriers. Unfortunately, this difficulty can lead to the selection of an instrument from a limited pool and thus may discourage obtaining the most appropriate choice of instruments.

Instrument modification is often a necessary addition to the instrument selection process. Standardized instruments may overlook individualized needs of specific patient populations. Therefore, modification, with permission, is often required. For example, increasing the size of the type font might be important for a study involving geriatric patients. The researcher should read the questionnaire from the perspective of the patient population involved in the study, and then evaluate any necessary changes. For example, in the study involving individuals with lower extremity paralysis, questions that used the word "walking" were modified. The distributor of the instrument should be contacted to ascertain how to make modifications with appropriate approval. The researcher does not want to interfere with the reliability or validity of the instrument and should consider this possibility when making any change.

When utilizing the Roy Adaptation Model as a theoretical framework for guiding nursing research and practice, the following step-by-step approach may be helpful in applying the model:

1. Identify a research question and conduct a comprehensive literature review contemplating the components of the theoretical framework and the potential study variables.
2. Evaluate the philosophical and conceptual congruence of the theoretical framework, nursing specialty, and practice domain.
3. Locate and refer to studies with similar research designs or content, which have utilized the Roy Adaptation Model as a conceptual framework.

4. Select and operationally define study variables.

5. Develop a schematic representation of the relationship between concepts within the theoretical framework and the study variables (Figure 4–2 is an example).

6. Review the research question and schematic overview with a mentor or colleague, to gain informed feedback.

7. Determine the method of study.

8. Select empirical instrumentation for variable measurement with quantitative research.

9. Refer to the Roy Adaptation Model for guidance throughout the study implementation, especially when crossroad decisions must be made.

10. Interpret the research findings within the context of the theoretical framework, comparing and contrasting the direction and relationship of the research outcome variables and the theoretical framework.

THE ROY ADAPTATION MODEL IN RESEARCH: THE BROADER PICTURE

In a recent critique of nursing theory, a noted author claimed, "A major failure of the grand theories was that they were not very useful in the scientific enterprise" (Bullough & Bullough, 1994, p. 75). The writer included Roy as the "most well-known of the California theorists" and described the moves to adopt the Roy model to structure nursing practice in several Canadian hospitals in the 1980s. There was no mention of nursing research using the Roy model. In the critique of grand theories in general, it was noted that they were seldom used in the research process. A recent review of 25 years of research based on the Roy Adaptation Model provides evidence to the contrary (Roy, Lauchner, Massey, & Carson, 1995; Roy, Pollock, et al., 1995). A comprehensive computerized search was conducted for all publications from January 1970 through December 1994, and included nine databases. The search identified 452 potential publications. Abstracts were hand-searched to screen for three criteria: (a) empirical work that explicitly identified the Roy Adaptation

Model as the theoretical underpinning of the research project; (b) a primary research report; and (c) journal publication, thesis, or dissertation. A final list of 188 research reports met the criteria to be included in a project of critical analysis and synthesis of Roy Adaptation Model research.

Of particular note in describing the broad picture of Roy Adaptation Model research are several observations from the first phase of the larger project, the retrieval of the research reports. First, the number of reported research studies has increased steadily in the 25-year period since the publication of the first theoretical article on the model in 1970. In fact, there has been a doubling of reports every three years; the most recent time frame, 1992 to 1994, showed over 100 studies. Second, there is evidence of programs of research by at least five investigators, or teams of investigators, who have three or more publications each on the same topic. Next, the areas of practice represented in the research range widely, utilizing samples from low-birth-weight infants in neonatal intensive care units to visually impaired elderly in rural Africa. The number of English-speaking journals publishing Roy Adaptation Model research is at least 46, and studies have come from eight different countries: United States, Canada, South Africa, Sweden, United Kingdom, Taiwan, Thailand, and the Netherlands. As to content, the studies represent all the major concepts of the Roy Adaptation Model and are focused on individuals and on groups, including research on applications in nursing education and nursing practice.

The identification of studies and the retrieval of research reports based on the Roy Adaptation Model is only one step in describing the broad picture of research based on the model. The major question of the model's contribution to nursing science can be addressed by the analysis and critique of this body of work. This project is being carried out by a team of investigators from the Boston Based Adaptation Research in Nursing Society (BBARNS). The central purpose of this project is to identify contributions to nursing science and to derive implications for nursing practice and for future theory development and research. The project is in its second year and has approximately one year to completion. This group of researchers has been working together for five years and formed a society to share scholarly interests and conduct selected common projects. Each of the investigators had been using the Roy Adaptation Model to guide individual work. One publication (Pollock, Frederickson, Carson, Massey, & Roy, 1994), a synthesis of findings from research of four original members of the society, showed that the research of several authors using the same model goes beyond the work of any one individual. Important theoretical and empirical relationships emerge when studies are viewed collectively. This collective view in turn facilitates the development of further theory and research.

SUMMARY

The development of knowledge for nursing practice is the goal of nursing research. The primary purpose of the Roy Adaptation Model is to contribute to the scientific discipline of nursing and nursing practice by directing research in understanding the basic life processes that foster health (the basic science of nursing), and in discovering how individuals cope with health and illness and the promotion of adaptive coping (the clinical science of nursing). Utilization of the Roy Adaptation Model when conducting nursing research is done for the purpose of further developing the basic science and/or the clinical science of nursing. The study presented in this chapter attempted to further explicate the clinical science of nursing. Scholarly knowledge development in the discipline of nursing is dependent on continued development, implementation, evaluation, and interpretation of model-based nursing research. Through scientific research, theoretical and empirical relationships will emerge, providing direction for research and theory growth and, ultimately, the development of nursing practice.

REFERENCES

Andrews, H., & Roy, C. (1986). *Essentials of the Roy Adaptation Model* (pp. 17–48). Norwalk, CT: Appleton-Century-Crofts.

Barone, S. (1993). Adaptation to spinal cord injury (Doctoral dissertation, Boston College). *Dissertation Abstracts International, 54,* 3547-B.

Boyle, A., Grap, M., Younger, J., & Thornby, D. (1991). Personality hardiness, ways of coping, social support and burnout in critical care nurses. *Journal of Advanced Nursing, 16*, 850-857.

Bullough, B., & Bullough, V. (Eds.). (1994). Nursing theory: History and critique. In *Nursing issues for the nineties and beyond* (pp. 64-82). New York: Springer.

Contrada, R. (1985). Type A behavior, hardiness, and the subjective and cardiovascular response to performance challenge. *Dissertation Abstracts International, 46,* 5-B 1733, (University Microfilms No. 85-15613).

Cyr, L. (1989). Sequelae of spinal cord injury after discharge from the initial rehabilitation program. *Rehabilitation Nursing, 14*(6), 326-329.

Derogatis, R. (1990). *Psychosocial adjustment to illness survey. Administration, scoring and procedures manual.* Baltimore: Clinical Psychometric Research.

Dew, M., Lynch, K., Ernst, J., Rosenthal, R., & Judd, C. (1985). A causal analysis of factors affecting adjustment to spinal cord injury. *Rehabilitation Psychology, 30*(1), 40-45.

Dittmar, S. (1989). *Rehabilitation nursing.* Baltimore: Mosby.

Driever, M. (1976). Theory of self concept. In Sr. C. Roy, *Introduction to nursing: An adaptation model* (pp. 169-79). Englewood Cliffs, NJ: Prentice-Hall.

Folkman, S., & Lazarus, R. (1980). An analysis of coping in a middle-aged community sample. *Journal of Health and Social Behavior, 21*, 219-39.

Folkman, S., & Lazarus, R. (1988). *Manual for the ways of coping questionnaire.* Palo Alto, CA: Consulting Psychologist Press.

Fuller, E. (1982). Selecting a clinical nursing problem for research. *Image: The Journal of Nursing Scholarship, 16*, 60-61.

Helson, H. (1964). *Adaptation level theory.* New York: Harper & Row.

Kobasa, S. (1979). Stressful life events, personality and health: An inquiry into hardiness. *Journal of Personality and Social Psychology, 37*(1), 1-11.

Lee, H. (1983). Analysis of a concept: Hardiness. *Oncology Nursing Forum, 10*(4), 32-35.

Lindeman, C., & Schantz, D. (1982). The research question. *Journal of Nursing Administration, 12*(1), 6-10.

Mateo, M., & Kirchhoff, K. (1991). *Conducting and using nursing research in the clinical setting.* Baltimore: Williams & Wilkins.

Norris, S., Campbell, L., & Brenhert, S. (1982). Nursing procedures and alteration in transcutaneous oxygen tension in premature infants. *Nursing Research, 31*, 330-36.

Pollock, S. (1986). Human responses to chronic illness: Physiologic and psychosocial adaptation. *Nursing Research, 35*(2), 90-95.

Pollock, S. (1989a). Adaptive responses to diabetes mellitus. *Western Journal of Nursing Research, 11,* 265-280.

Pollock, S. (1989b). The hardiness characteristic: A motivating factor in adaptation. *Advances Nursing Research, 11,* 53-62.

Pollock, S., & Duffy, M. (1990). The health-related hardiness scale: Development and psychometric analysis. *Nursing Research, 39*(4), 218-222.

Pollock, S., Frederickson, K., Carson, M., Massey, V., & Roy, C. (1994). Contributions to nursing science: Synthesis of findings from adaptation model research. *Scholarly Inquiry for Nursing Practice, 8*(4), 361-72.

Riehl, J., & Roy, C. (1980). *Conceptual models for nursing practice* (2nd ed. pp. 106-142). New York: Appleton-Century-Crofts.

Roy, Sr. C. (1967). Role cues and mothers of hospitalized children. *Nursing Research, 16*(2), 178-82.

Roy, Sr. C. (1976). *Introduction to nursing: An adaptation model.* Englewood Cliffs, NJ: Prentice-Hall.

Roy, Sr. C. (1987). Response to "Needs of spouses of surgical patients: A conceptualization within the Roy Adaptation Model." *Scholarly Inquiry for Nursing Practice: An International Journal, 1*(1), 45-50.

Roy, Sr. C. (1988). An explication of the philosophical assumptions of the Roy Adaptation Model. *Nursing Science Quarterly, 1*(1), 26-34.

Roy, Sr. C. (1990). Theorist's response to "Strengthening the Roy Adaptation Model through conceptual clarification." *Nursing Science Quarterly, 3*(2), 64-66.

Roy, Sr. C., & Andrews, H. (1991). *The Roy Adaptation Model: The definitive statement.* Norwalk, CT: Appleton & Lange.

Roy, Sr. C., Lauchner, K., Massey, V., & Carson, M. (1995). *Contributions to nursing science: Research based on the Roy Adaptation Model.* Paper presented at the International Nursing Congress, Athens, Greece.

Roy, Sr. C., Pollock, S., Carson, M., Lauchner, K., Massey, V., Whetsell, M., & Frederickson, K. (1995). *Contributions to nursing science: 25th anniversary of the Roy Adaptation Model of nursing.* Athens, Greece: Monograph in Progress.

Smith, P., Hamilton, B., & Granger, C. (1990). Functional independence measure decision tree. *The FONE FIM.* Buffalo, NY: Research Foundation of the State University of New York.

von Bertalanffy, L. (1968). *General systems theory.* New York: Braziller.

Section III

Blueprints for Education

5

The Neuman Systems Model in Nursing Education

Victoria Strickland Seng, Rosalie Mirenda, and Lois W. Lowry

At UCLA, in 1970, I first introduced a wholistic teaching and practice model that would assist graduate nursing students in synthesizing course content with clinical specialties and would later guide their clinical practice in a wholistic manner.

As illustrated in this chapter, the futuristic model concepts are readily adaptable to various levels of nurse educational programming. For example, to complement the baccalaureate program shared here, a Neuman-based Master's level program is being developed at Neumann College. Also, for over a decade a nurse practitioner program has been in place at the California State University, Fresno.

The Neuman work continues its development worldwide as the model is applied in a wide variety of levels of nursing and interdisciplinary cross-cultural education and practice programs.

Betty Neuman

IMPLEMENTATION OF THE MODEL

The Neuman Systems Model provides a comprehensive outline for the subject matter that comprises the practice discipline of nursing. The model diagram (see Figure 5-1) demonstrates application of the model to an individual; however, Neuman (1995) noted that the model principles, concepts, and processes can be applied to families, groups, communities, and social issues as well. This chapter focuses on use of the model in two undergraduate programs: (a) the associate degree program at Cecil Community College in North East, Maryland, and (b) the baccalaureate program at Neumann College in Aston, Pennsylvania.

Baccalaureate Degree

During the early 1970s, a decision was made at Neumann College. The nursing faculty would develop a curriculum that depended on a nursing conceptual model to guide the selection of content and the planning of learning experiences. Established in March 1965, Neumann College, a Catholic college in the Franciscan tradition, offers a Christian education based on the concept that the individual's physical, emotional, spiritual, and intellectual growth occurs through the complementarity and interrelationships of these human dimensions. As Neumann College ("the College") was realizing its beginning, members of the Sisters of St. Francis of Philadelphia urged the establishment of a collegiate nursing program. All possessed a singular commitment to develop a liberal-arts-based, integrated baccalaureate program in nursing that would be noted for its excellence. The nursing faculty focused on their interest and desire to ensure a nursing program that maintained consistency with the College's philosophy and mission and that centered on the growing body of nursing knowledge. Faculty endorsed a commitment to the early engagement of professional nursing students in the discovery of connections between and among education, practice, and research.

Nursing's metaparadigm (consisting of the four core concepts of person, environment, health, and nursing), coupled with the College's and the nursing faculty's value for human wholeness and person–environment interaction, rendered liberal education and the selection of a systems-based conceptual model of nursing critically

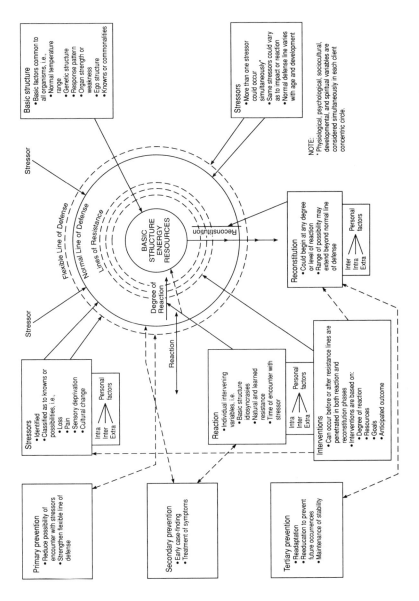

Figure 5–1. The Neuman Systems Model. Original diagram copyright © 1970 by Betty Neuman.

important in the development of the professional nurse. The decision to adopt the Neuman Systems Model was made in the Spring of 1976, after faculty had engaged in a period of critical analysis of current and available nursing models for their relevance and applicability to the program and to the faculty's beliefs about the discipline of nursing. The Neuman model met the faculty's expectations because the model identifies a systems perspective of the metaparadigm of nursing and supports the views that nursing involves primary, secondary, and tertiary levels of prevention as interventions and that the client system can be an individual or group (Neuman, 1982, 1989, 1995). Faculty recognized that the Neuman Systems Model would provide the scope, complexity, and clinical usefulness vital to nursing and the development of its future theoretical structures (Mirenda, 1995).

Associate Degree

Cecil County, in northeast Maryland, mandated that Cecil Community College begin a nursing program following completion of a needs assessment in 1980. Lois W. Lowry was hired, in January 1981, to develop the program and serve as its first director. At that time, Lowry was deeply engaged in learning about the efficacy of nursing models as a doctoral student at the University of Pennsylvania. To fulfill course requirements, Lowry had selected the Neuman Systems Model for an in-depth analysis and evaluation. Through this intensive study, Lowry realized that the Neuman Systems Model could appropriately guide curriculum development and provide a comprehensive structure for the entire process of educational programming. Heretofore, the Neuman Systems Model had been used by several baccalaureate programs as a framework for curriculum, but had not been used at the associate degree level anywhere in the United States. Use of the model would create a *nursing* emphasis for teaching concepts and processes (as opposed to the traditional medical approach) and would provide additional preparation for associate degree students continuing on for a baccalaureate degree (Lowry, 1986). The program at Cecil Community College became the first to use the Neuman Systems Model as the conceptual framework for associate level curricula.

PHILOSOPHICAL RELATIONSHIP OF THE MODEL TO THE SETTING AND USER

Theoretical Underpinnings

The Neuman Systems Model views the open system of the client as an integrated whole that must be considered in totality when examining the impact of environmental stressors on the system and selecting preventions as interventions. Neuman (1995) attributes key theoretical influences on the model to the Gestalt views of Teilhard de Chardin (1955), Cornu (1957), and Edelson (1970), and to Selye's (1950) conceptualization of stress. Other theorists were referenced as influencing the development of the Neuman Systems Model: the dynamic view of systems held by von Bertalanffy (1968), Emery (1969), and Putt (1978), and the levels of prevention derived from Caplan (1964). When implementing the model in educational settings, these theoretical influences must be carefully considered.

Baccalaureate Degree.   Nursing faculty at Neumann College ascribe to a wholistic (Neumann College's use of the spelling "wholistic" is in keeping with the preference of the college and the primary source; see Neuman, 1980, 1989, 1995) view of individuals, health, and nursing, and they believe that individuals exist as complex systems composed of interdependent components. The wholistic and systems perspective of individuals applies to any client system, faculty, learner, health, and nursing.

The curriculum of the Neumann College nursing program reflects the worldview expressed through its selected conceptual model of nursing, the Neuman Systems Model. The Neuman Systems Model is classified as a systems model (Neuman, 1982; Riehl & Roy, 1974) and emulates a reciprocal interaction worldview (Fawcett, 1989, 1995) as exemplified in the definition of person as an interacting, open client system consisting of a dynamic composite of interrelated physiological, psychological, sociocultural, developmental, and spiritual variables (Neuman, 1980, 1985). The model embodies elements of both persistence and change, the attributes of the reciprocal interaction worldview (Fawcett, 1995). Neuman (1995) wrote:

The client is an interacting open system in total interface with both internal and external environmental forces of stressors; the client is in constant change, with reciprocal environmental interaction, moving either toward a dynamic state of stability (wellness) or toward one of illness in varying degrees. (p. 12)

From its description and adoption in 1976, the curriculum has remained consistent with both the systems perspective and the reciprocal interaction worldview expressed in the Neuman Systems Model (Neuman, 1972, 1982, 1989, 1995). Persons, both in terms of clients and learners, are viewed as wholistic and interacting human beings. Just as nursing interventions are taught to be related to the dynamic organization of the interdependent parts of the whole affecting the client, faculty assist students in analyzing the reciprocal influence of life experience and the self, and provide opportunities for students to learn the interactive nature of nursing science with other sciences.

Associate Degree.   In the Cecil Community College program, the faculty readily accepted the model's concepts: stress/adaptation; wholism; and primary, secondary, and tertiary care. The Neuman Systems Model served as the source for the program's philosophy and objectives, which incorporated the dynamic system of the person in constant interaction with environmental stressors that have the potential for creating illness (Lowry, 1986).

Purpose of Model

According to Neuman (1995), "the purpose of the model is to help nurses organize the nursing field within a broad systems perspective as a logical way of dealing with its growing complexity" (p. 22). The model greatly assists education, functioning as a tool for faculty in structuring the curriculum, and for students in organizing their expanding knowledge base.

Relationship of the Model to Baccalaureate Education.   Mirenda (1986a) points out that the Neuman Systems Model was used by the faculty to define the unique focus of the curriculum as the relationship and interaction occurring between the nurse and the client system as the latter responds to stressors in the environment. The overall purpose of this program is stated as: The promotion of learning how to determine and provide primary, secondary, and tertiary levels of prevention to assist the client system in retaining, attaining, or maintaining an optimal level of wellness (Neumann College Nursing Program, 1984). The concepts and theories based on the Neuman Systems Model, and fundamental to the nursing program's design for curriculum, work through nursing intervention to provide essential assistance to a client system in maintaining its integrity and adapting to external and internal environmental stressors.

The Neumann College Nursing Program faculty attest to the contribution of the Neuman Systems Model to curriculum. The model was selected because of its strong wholistic, integrated, interdisciplinary approach. This approach within the health care system milieu gives new dimensions to the nursing curriculum and to nursing practice. The model is attuned to the thrust of modern nursing as a unique but interdependent care profession.

Relationship of the Model to Associate Degree Education.   The Neuman Systems Model serves as the source for Cecil Community College's philosophical framework as well as the foundation for the program objectives. Lowry (1989) noted that the curriculum emphasized the wholistic view of the client, encompassing Neuman's five variables in a constantly active relationship with each other and with stressors from all areas of the environment. The disequilibrium created by the stressors established the need for nursing intervention through the three prevention levels of the Neuman Systems Model. The model serves as an organizational tool for all nursing courses with objectives derived from the concepts and subconcepts in a progressively complex manner. Figure 5-2 depicts the Neuman Systems Model at Cecil Community College.

Concepts and Subconcepts

Concepts in the Neuman Systems Model address the client/client system, environment, health, and nursing interventions. The client/client system includes the core or basic structure, the line of resistance, the normal and flexible lines of defense, and five variables (physiological, psychological, sociocultural, developmental, and spiritual). The environment consists of internal, external, and

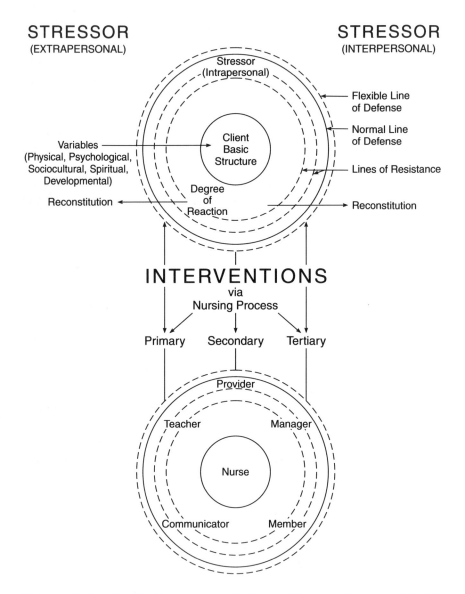

Figure 5–2. Cecil Community College, Neuman Systems Model. [From Lowry, L. W., & Green, G. H. (1989). Four Neuman-based associate degree nursing programs: Brief description and evaluation. In B. Neuman (Ed.), *The Neuman Systems Model* (2nd ed., p. 288). Norwalk, CT: Appleton & Lange. Used with permission.]

created components with intrapersonal, interpersonal, and extrapersonal stressors. Health is equated with wellness and viewed in terms of entropy and negentropy energy flow. Nursing is comprised of three preventions as intervention (primary, secondary, and tertiary) guided by a three-step nursing process (nursing diagnosis, nursing goals, and nursing outcomes; Neuman, 1995).

All the concepts and subconcepts typically are included in the educational implementation of the model within the curricula for associate and baccalaureate programs. The concepts are introduced in first-level courses and explored in subsequent courses. The emphasis placed on each concept or subconcept varies according to the course content and client population cared for in each course. Students also progress in the examination of the increasingly complex interactions among the concepts of the model as they advance through the curriculum. The final courses emphasize integration of all components of the model in a wholistic manner.

Baccalaureate Program. The Neumann College nursing curriculum reflects the use of the Neuman Systems Model's major concepts and their linkages throughout the courses and the course objectives. Study of Neuman's description of the four major concepts of the metaparadigm of nursing reveals relationships and linkages between or among (a) client and environment; (b) health and nursing; (c) client–environment, health, and nursing; (d) primary prevention and wellness retention; (e) secondary prevention and wellness attainment; and (f) tertiary prevention and wellness maintenance (Fawcett, 1995; Neuman, 1995).

The key concepts from the Neuman Systems Model and their linkages assist Neumann College's nursing faculty in identifying the areas of emphasis for the curriculum. These concepts also follow the metaparadigm of nursing. The client system as individual, family, or community incorporates a composite of five variables (physiological, psychological, sociocultural, developmental, and spiritual), a flexible line of defense, lines of resistance, and a basic energy structure. Environmental stressors are classified as internal and external and arise from intra-, extra-, and interpersonal, familial, or community sources. Wellness is viewed as optimal system stability, and variances from wellness are caused by stressors that penetrate the system's lines of defense. The profession of nursing is concerned with all the variables affecting the system's response to stressors and with the provision of primary, secondary, and tertiary levels of prevention (Neuman, 1982, 1989, 1995).

The content map, course descriptions, and course syllabi provide evidence of detailed use of these major concepts of the Neuman model to organize and sequence content. Students begin the courses in the nursing major in the second semester of the sophomore level. The first major course introduces students to the discipline of nursing, its metaparadigm, and the role of the nurse as one of the major health care providers in the U.S. health care system. In the presentation of the relationship between research and the development of nursing theory and practice, Neuman's conceptual model is introduced as a systems model and a viable framework for the professional study of an approach to the practice of nursing. The model is described and its component parts are examined for individual and interdependent characteristics. The nursing process format (Neuman, 1982), which operationalizes the model, is introduced and used as the scientific method of problem solving applied to the practice of nursing.

At the junior level, the first clinical nursing course focuses on health assessment of client systems, individuals, families, and communities. Identification of stressors, as they relate to physiological, psychological, sociocultural, developmental, and spiritual factors that pose a risk to the health of the client system, is emphasized. The concept of primary prevention is expanded at this level to include student experiences in community settings such as schools. Students are involved in both health assessment and health education, in keeping with Neuman's view of health promotion as a component of the primary prevention modality. Secondary prevention is introduced at the junior level and further developed at the senior level.

Senior-level students utilize the nursing process with individuals and groups who have developed signs of reaction to stressors and require secondary preventions. Students help client systems use internal and external resources to reduce reactions to the stressor and work toward stability. Tertiary prevention is also developed in the senior year. At this level, student use the nursing process to work with clients in planning and implementing approaches that will maximize and maintain optimal wellness levels for the client systems that have experienced a health crisis where some degree of reconstitution or stability has occurred after treatment. Nursing interventions focus on strengthening the lines of defense and on education to amend the client's optimal stability or wellness level.

As a curriculum structure, the Neuman Systems Model provides both conceptual and practical means of designing and organizing a curricular sequence. The sequence of content and learning activity inferred from Neuman's explanation of the Neuman Systems Model—its concepts, linkages, and relationships—is handled within a systems perspective. While identifying each component in an orderly manner for the purpose of developing greater understanding and insight into the character of the nursing practice suggested by the Neuman model, the learner is reminded that the concepts are interdependent: they link with one another to form the whole of nursing.

Associate Degree Program.   At Cecil Community College, in the first semester, faculty present the model, its main concepts, and the nursing process. Elderly clients serve as the clinical focus, and students identify stressors and work toward achieving proficiency initially in secondary prevention as intervention as well as in basic nursing skills. During the second semester, the emphasis shifts to adult clients across the lifespan who are experiencing simple and complex stressors. Students begin to provide total client care through secondary and tertiary prevention strategies. This semester also highlights implementation of the model with psychiatric clients.

The third semester shifts the client focus to developmental concerns of families, by examining infants, children, adolescents, and expectant women. Students concentrate on primary and secondary preventions. The final semester includes clients at all developmental levels who are experiencing complex stressors requiring intervention from the three preventions. Emphasis is placed on implementation of the model using a wholistic approach (Lowry & Green, 1989).

Concept Definitions and Relationships

Client/Client System.   The client/client system consists of a dynamic open system of concentric circles progressing outward from the core or basic structure through the lines of resistance, normal line of defense, and flexible line of defense. The client/client system may be comprised of individuals, families, groups, communities, or social issues, and it encompasses the physiological, psychological, sociocultural, developmental, and spiritual variables. The core or basic structure contains factors that are typical of all human beings. The lines of resistance encircle the core and protect it when stressors penetrate the lines of defense. The normal line of defense constitutes the client's normal wellness state, and the flexible line of defense serves as the buffer or first line of defense against stressors.

In addition to the basic structure or core, each client/client system possesses five types of variables that establish its uniqueness through the degree of their development and interaction. The physiological variable consists of the body's structure and functioning. Affective and cognitive functions are identified as the psychological variable. Social and cultural influences jointly comprise the sociocultural variable. The developmental variable refers to considerations related to development throughout the lifespan. The spiritual variable constitutes the spiritual beliefs and values of the client/client system (Neuman, 1995).

Environment. The environment refers to the context within which the client/client system exists; it includes the created environment. Every internal and external factor interacting with the client/client system makes up the environment. The internal environment encompasses all influencing factors within the perimeter of the client/client system; the external environment contains those factors beyond the client/client system's boundaries. The created environment refers to the subconscious formulation of a milieu based on the perceptions of the actual internal and external environments, which allows the client/client system to function comfortably.

Stressors are factors in the environment that positively or negatively influence the client/client system. Intrapersonal stressors occur within the boundaries of the client/client system as a part of the internal environment. Interpersonal and extrapersonal stressors exist in the external environment beyond the perimeter of the client/client system. Interpersonal stressors occur proximally, and extrapersonal stressors occur distally. All three types of stressors may be included in the created environment (Neuman, 1995).

Health. The Neuman Systems Model places health or wellness on a continuum with optimal stability of the client/client system (negentropy) anchoring one end and illness (entropy) placed at the other end. The energy flow between the client/client system and the environment determines the position on the continuum. When the response to stressors requires less energy than is being produced, then a state of negentropy exists. Entropy occurs when the amount of energy necessary to respond to stressors exceeds that which is being generated (Neuman, 1995).

Nursing. Nursing as a profession functions to assist the client/client system in its quest for stability. Primary prevention as intervention focuses on retaining wellness and on the flexible line of defense. When stressors penetrate the flexible and normal lines of defense, secondary prevention as intervention concentrates on fortifying the internal lines of resistance in order to regain wellness or attain reconstitution. Reconstitution refers to the return and maintenance of a level of stability for the system. During reconstitution, tertiary prevention as intervention serves to preserve the system's stability, whether at previous or adjusted levels (Neuman, 1995).

Baccalaureate Program Definitions.   Neumann College utilizes the definitions of concepts as delineated by Neuman (1982, 1989, 1995).

Associate Degree Definitions.   At Cecil Community College, the concepts were defined as Neuman (1982) defined them. Faculty concurred with the basic definitions, but expanded the definitions of the physiological, psychological, sociocultural, and spiritual variables to incorporate several subconcepts. The physiological variable subconcepts encompassed safety, comfort, mobility, nutrition, elimination, oxygenation, circulation, and sexuality. Subconcepts for the psychological variable addressed the cognitive and affective domains and were identified as interpersonal relationships, communication, thought processes, crisis, and self-concept. The focus for the sociocultural variable subconcepts included family, ethnic background, environment, occupation, hobbies, and recreation. Religious beliefs, morals, ethics, and values comprised the subconcepts for the spiritual variable (Lowry, 1986).

At Cecil Community College, the model influenced and shaped the political and social environment of the institution by creating the culture for the nursing program. The model provided a structure, a vocabulary, and goals that set the standard for the program. Then faculty and students lived up to the challenge (Lowry & Jopp, 1989).

Structure of Model

The Neuman Systems Model, originally designed for use with graduate students, employs a systems approach to organize information. Commonalities within the client/client system are acknowledged by the core or basic structure, and differences are recognized through the variables. The concentric circles comprising the client/client system's core, lines of resistance, normal line of defense, and flexible line of defense demonstrate the complexity of the system and its response to stressors in the environment. The client/client system's constant interaction with and definition of its environment emphasize the dynamic nature of the model's structure. Placing health on a continuum and focusing nursing on preventions as intervention allow for individual differences in the levels of health among client/client systems and the activities necessary for achieving stability of the system. The strong emphasis on the wholistic view ensures inclusion of the entire client/client system when implementing the model. The structure (a) provides the scope necessary to address a large knowledge base in education when establishing curricula and (b) allows easy manipulation of the knowledge by students at all levels.

Baccalaureate Degree Program. The curriculum sequence related to the learning of major concepts and subconcepts is inferred from the organization and description of nursing and nursing practice as delineated by the Neuman Systems Model. The faculty's decision to teach primary prevention first, so that secondary and tertiary preventions when learned and applied could be accompanied by primary preventions as appropriate, stemmed specifically from Neuman's (1995) expressed thoughts:

> *The model format for prevention as intervention provides an intervention typology. First considered is primary prevention as intervention. This modality is used for primary prevention as wellness*

retention. . . . Ideally, primary prevention is considered concomitant with secondary and tertiary preventions as interventions. (p. 33)

The nursing program faculty at Neumann College utilize systems theory and the Neuman Systems Model to introduce and describe the discipline of nursing and the role of the nurse as one of the major health care providers. The faculty developed a sequence of courses and broad areas of content consistent with the Neuman Systems Model and the assumptions inherent within the model as identified by Neuman in her conversations with faculty and later listed in her publications.

Associate Degree Program. At Cecil Community College, the Neuman Systems Model provided the structures for placement of material in the program. The program's philosophy and objectives were derived from the model, and, as noted earlier, the content in the courses was organized in a manner that allowed progressive integration of the model by the students (Lowry, 1986). For the educational process, the Neuman Systems Model provided a structure that included student, faculty, and client, as shown in Figure 5-3. Each segment of the structure represents an open system that is interacting with other open systems. The student achieves the roles of care provider, teacher, and manager of care. Faculty fulfill the roles of teacher, advisor, counselor, and role model. Students use primary, secondary, and tertiary preventions as intervention to interact with the patient system. Stressors impact students; faculty seek to establish or influence stability (homeostasis) for students. The structure of the Neuman Systems Model is viewed as functional and practical for nursing education (Lowry, 1986).

Underlying Assumptions

For her model, Neuman (1985, pp. 20–21) states ten basic assumptions that she now also views as propositions:

1. Although each individual client or group constituting a client system is unique, each system is also unique because each system is a composite of common known factors or

innate characteristics within a normal, given range of response contained within a basic structure.

2. Many known, unknown, and universal environmental stressors exist. Each differs in its potential for disturbing a client's
usual stability level, or normal line of defense. The particular
interrelationships of client variables—physiological, psychological, sociocultural, developmental, and spiritual—at any
point in time can affect the degree to which a client is pro-
tected by the flexible line of defense against possible reaction
to a single stressor or a combination of stressors.

3. Each individual client/client system has evolved a normal
range of response to the environment that is referred to as
the normal line of defense, or the usual wellness/stability
state. The range of response changes over time through coping with diverse stress encounters. The normal line of defense can be used as a standard from which to measure
health deviation.

4. When the cushioning, accordion-like effect of the flexible line
of defense is no longer capable of protecting the client/client
system against an environmental stressor, the stressor breaks
through the normal line of defense. The interrelationships of
variables—physiological, psychological, sociocultural, developmental, and spiritual—determine the nature and degree of
system reaction or the possible reaction to the stressor.

5. The client, whether in a state of wellness or illness, is a dynamic composite of the interrelationships of variables—
physiological, psychological, sociocultural, developmental,
and spiritual. Wellness is on a continuum of available energy
to support the system in an optimal state of system stability.

6. Implicit within each client system are internal resistance factors known as lines of resistance, which function to stabilize
and return the client to the usual wellness state (normal line
of defense) or possibly to a higher level of stability following
an environmental stressor reaction.

7. Primary prevention relates to general knowledge that is applied in client assessment and intervention to identify and
reduce or mitigate possible or actual risk factors associated

with environmental stressors, in order to prevent possible reaction.

8. Secondary prevention relates to symptomatology following a reaction to stressors, appropriate ranking of intervention priorities, and treatment to reduce their noxious effects.

9. Tertiary prevention relates to the adjustive processes taking place as reconstitution begins and maintenance factors move the client back in a circular manner toward primary prevention.

10. The client as a system is in dynamic, constant energy exchange with the environment.

Given these assumptions or propositions, implementation of the model requires that leaders in an educational program obtain agreement to and acceptance of the assumptions and the model among all the faculty. Both primary and secondary sources verify that the philosophical claims and assumptions on which the Neuman Systems Model is based include beliefs about person–environment, health or wellness, stability, change, and nursing (Fawcett, 1995; Marriner, 1986; Neuman, 1995).

Baccalaureate Degree Program.   The explicit philosophic claims of the Neumann College nursing program curriculum include beliefs about (a) person–environment, in terms of both the client system and the beliefs inferred about the learner and the learner-environment from Neuman's view of person; (b) health and wellness, and inferences about students' learning from Neuman's view of health; and (c) nursing and inferences made about education from Neuman's view of nursing. The philosophical claims of the Neumann College nursing program are operationalized, and inferences about the learner, the learner-environment, students' learning, and education are made to be consistent with the underlying assumptions and claims of the Neuman Systems Model (see Appendix A).

Associate Degree Program.   At Cecil Community College, the faculty recognized that a nursing model would provide a nursing perspective rather than a traditional medical perspective for instruction, and they identified four assumptions related to use of nursing models:

1. Models provide a structure for organizing curricular content for students.

2. Models introduce relevant nursing concepts and help illustrate the relationships among them.

3. If broad in scope, models remain adaptable as future changes occur in the health care system.

4. Models provide a guide for nursing practice—that is, concepts taught in the classroom apply equally well to clinical practice settings. (Lowry & Jopp, 1989, pp. 73-74)

The faculty found the Neuman Systems Model compatible with their assumptions and philosophy, and the model was adopted.

PRACTICAL ASPECTS OF MODEL IMPLEMENTATION

Determining the Fit of the Neuman Systems Model to Education

The conceptual model of nursing selected for curriculum construction provides the map for all curricular matters. Such a model for a nursing educational program reflects the school's philosophical setting, educational setting, the community it serves, the students who enroll and attend, and the characteristics of the faculty. These characteristics include the faculty's beliefs about nursing and people (Scales, 1985). When selecting the Neuman Systems Model for implementation in the educational setting, faculty must compare their program philosophy and assumptions with those of the model to determine how well they fit together.

Baccalaureate Program. The Neumann College nursing faculty utilized a strategy for developing the curriculum that included the articulation of a philosophy of curriculum, a conceptual model of nursing (specifically, the Neuman Systems Model), and beliefs about learning. This combination of philosophy, subject matter, and beliefs about learning articulated by the Neumann College nursing faculty was recently analyzed and evaluated through the application of a strategy developed to determine compatibility among these three essential components of curriculum development. Evidence in this study indicates curriculum compatibility and congruence with systems thinking and the Neuman Systems Model (Mirenda, 1995).

The faculty beliefs about the discipline of nursing that were determined to be congruent with the Neuman Systems Model include:

1. A systems perspective of persons, health, and nursing is critical.
2. Persons exist as complex systems composed of interdependent variables.
3. Nursing is dynamic and is involved with health promotion and with therapeutic and rehabilitative care.
4. Nursing is concerned with individuals, families, and community.
5. Nursing is in the throes of gaining recognized professional status.
6. Nursing necessitates collaboration in multiple systems.

Associate Degree Program.   Faculty at Cecil Community College compared the program's philosophy and assumptions with those of the Neuman Systems Model and found close correlation between the two. Fit of the model could be further determined by internalization of the model by the faculty. Lowry and Jopp (1989) outlined a number of tasks and strategies that were focused on that internalization. Prior to beginning intensive work with the model, faculty worked to thoroughly review the literature, develop and define concepts and subconcepts, and determine the scope of the model within the curricular structure and clinical experiences. In the associate degree program at Cecil Community College, emphasis was placed on secondary prevention as intervention, in accordance with guidelines established for the scope of practice for the associate degree graduate in 1981. Completion of these tasks confirmed the fit of the model with the program. Over time, emphasis on the preventions as intervention has changed in response to the broadening scope of associate education.

Client Populations

The client/client system in the Neuman Systems Model may be defined as an individual, family, group, community, or social issue. The broad definition for this concept provides flexibility for faculty in planning the curriculum.

Baccalaureate Program. Nursing faculty at Neumann College selected clinical settings for the opportunities they offered for learning and for providing primary, secondary, and tertiary preventions by the students. The clinical settings utilized by the nursing program vary from large medical centers to local community health care agencies and clients' homes. These agencies, located in three states and six different counties, reflect populations with a fairly wide range of ethnic and economic diversity. Regardless of the clinical area, students utilize the Neumann College Nursing Process Tool, based on the Neuman Systems Model, as the assessment intervention tool with client systems (individuals and groups) in communities reflective of varied cultures (e.g., migrant worker populations and the African American, Amish, Asian, and Hispanic communities).

Associate Degree Program. Generally, faculty begin by focusing on the client as an individual, an approach that allows students to master the variables and lines of resistance and defense for one client before expanding the client system to include broader groups. Expansion of the concept generally follows the pattern of adding families with maternal–child content, groups with mental health content, communities with community health content, and social issues with leadership and trends courses.

Cecil Community College followed this pattern by introducing the model and focusing on the aging adult client in the first level, and adding the adult and mental health client/client systems in the second level. The client system as family was introduced in the third level. The fourth level provided an opportunity for students to synthesize their knowledge of the client/client system (Lowry, 1986).

The client/client system can also be applied to the education process itself, with faculty and students each functioning as client systems. As Figure 5-3 shows, the curriculum model at Cecil Community College depicts each component as an open system

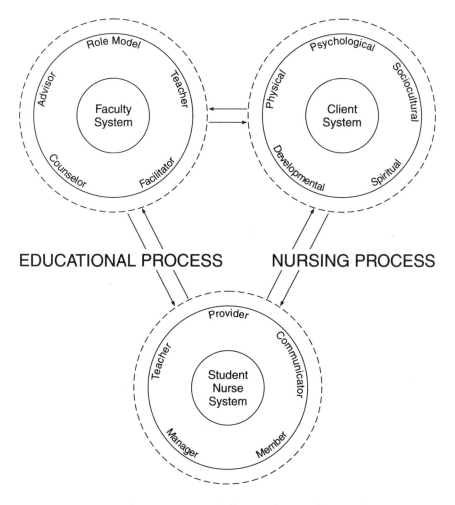

EDUCATIONAL PROCESS   NURSING PROCESS

Figure 5–3.   Cecil Community College: The Student as the Center of the System. [From Lowry, L. W., & Green, G. H. (1989). Four Neuman-based associate degree nursing programs: Brief description and evaluation. In B. Neuman (Ed.), *The Neuman Systems Model* (2nd ed., p. 299). Norwalk, CT: Appleton & Lange. Used with permission.]

interacting with the other persons in the system for the purpose of teaching students to provide primary, secondary, and tertiary care. Further, the educational process is described as a system in this way. Faculty, students, resources, and clinical agencies constitute inputs into the system. The teaching/learning process illustrates the throughput. The feedback loop, represented by tests, papers, care plans, clinical evaluations, and output, is expressed as either passing or failing. If failing occurs, the student reenters the system at the throughput through the feedback loop.

Preparing Faculty, Students, and Staff for Implementation of the Neuman Systems Model

Preparing faculty, students, and staff for implementation actually begins with selection of the model and development of the curriculum using the model. Strategies mentioned for assisting in the selection of the model also apply to preparing to implement the model.

Baccalaureate Program. The preparation of all involved at Neumann College for implementation of the nursing curriculum based on the Neuman Systems Model included the development of several conditions that may have contributed to its initial and ongoing success. These conditions were:

1. A strong commitment, on the part of the leadership of the college's nursing program and a core group of faculty, to a theoretically based curriculum.
2. A formal, systematic faculty orientation to the curriculum as developed and used, to ensure continuity and improvement of the theory-based approach to the curriculum.
3. Institutional support for the pioneering work done by the faculty, in terms of financial resources, library acquisitions, consultation, and curriculum evaluation.
4. The faculty's strong valuing of a systems-based approach to curriculum development and the view that curriculum development is a rigorous and scholarly effort.
5. Early and continued personal contact with Betty Neuman. This contact has fostered and nurtured the commitment to

implement and maintain the curriculum based on the Neuman Systems Model even though forces exist that mitigate against this persistence, such as emphasis on the medical model, use of the North American Nursing Diagnosis Association (NANDA) taxonomy in nursing, and concerns that integration represents an overly difficult and complex issue for curriculum.

Associate Degree Program. At Cecil Community College, the faculty spent many hours talking and listening to one another's interpretations of their perceptions of the Neuman Systems Model's definitions and propositions. They agreed among themselves on amplified definitions of some of the constructs. Specific tasks were divided among the faculty, and efforts were made to match individuals to their own areas of interest. Team-building activities were initiated when differences in commitment to implementation arose, and attention was given to values clarification in informal faculty work sessions. During these sessions, paradigm shifts were encouraged through use of creativity and risk taking. Timetables were recorded to ensure tracking of immediate and long-range plans, and one member of the team maintained notes of discussions to ensure documentation. Faculty were also encouraged to keep logs of ideas between sessions. Networking was established with other programs using the model (Lowry & Jopp, 1989). Dialogue between the faculties of Cecil Community College and Neumann College resulted in an articulated program.

Complexity of the Model and Implementation

If a conceptual model of nursing is to provide guidelines to construct a curriculum, faculty must discover a model that is sufficiently broad in scope that it can serve as a basis for the educational design and process (Fawcett, 1995). Because nursing is considered a practice discipline, faculty must be concerned with the model's adequacy for clinical situations encountered by nurses as a result of current, common, and geographical health care needs and settings (Donley, 1989; Fawcett, 1995). A conceptual model that is broad in scope will achieve four tasks:

1. The model should reveal the focus of the curriculum to be designed and the purposes to be fulfilled by the educational process.
2. The general nature and sequence of the content to be delineated should be identified.
3. Clues for settings in which the education occurs should be provided, along with student characteristics related to their preparation, background, attitude, and types of learning required.
4. The teaching–learning strategies to be utilized to enhance the learning required should be identified (Fawcett, 1995).

The Neuman Systems Model encompasses a broad scope. The model serves as an umbrella, with each spoke representing a concept. Each concept must be developed and linked to other concepts to create courses. Neuman (1995) noted that "earlier the model was criticized as being too broad; now this quality has become a major reason for increasing acceptance of the model and its proven utility" (p. 22).

The Neuman Systems Model, accompanied by learning theories and the program's philosophy, provides the framework necessary for constructing a curriculum. The model's overall open structure allows faculty to be creative in teaching content and process, thereby generating excitement when implementing it in education. The model user links specific information taught in courses with the model concepts. Betty Neuman encourages individuals to use and interpret the model creatively.

Baccalaureate Program. By examining available models for their breadth, the nursing faculty at Neumann College identified and selected the Neuman Systems Model for its provision of a basic structure for the curriculum; a system for classifying the knowledge, skill, and values of the discipline of nursing; and a way of ordering facts into a system that organizes subject matter into levels of functions in systems. The model further showed the relationships in the content considered essential for nursing and identified the goal of nursing. Neuman's model also depicted harmony of objectives and content with the College's philosophy and objectives, guided the development of instructional methodologies, and provided a schema for evaluation.

Associate Degree Program. The program at Cecil Community College was new under Lowry's administration. She determined that the model would be used as the conceptual framework for the program and then selected faculty to join in developing the curriculum. The fact that the Neuman Systems Model uses clear language and a vocabulary that is understood by lay persons proved a plus. People (faculty) understood the meaning of stress and adaptation; individuals, families, and communities as open systems; and the statement that too much stress breaks down one's health. Faculty readily accepted the utility of a model with such easily understood concepts. Models that avoid jargon are more user-friendly and more likely to be accepted.

Faculty at Cecil Community College implemented the model over a two-year period. Definition of terms, drafting of the curriculum, and development of the first-semester courses were accomplished during the first three months. The first year of the program was taught in the next nine months. The second year followed a similar pattern: course development during the summer, with implementation of the courses occurring in the academic year.

Accessibility of Experts

Nursing education programs interested in implementing the Neuman Systems Model at the associate, baccalaureate, and graduate levels can readily access expert assistance. The Neuman Systems Trustees Group, Inc., provides the names and addresses of trustees and associate members, and describes their expertise. A newsletter is mailed periodically, and the trustees sponsor international symposia on a biannual basis. Betty Neuman frequently provides direct consultation as well as the twenty-two trustees.

Baccalaureate Program. During the period of time devoted to initial curriculum development, little existed in the literature to assist the Neumann College faculty in systematically developing a curriculum that proved attentive to internal order and consistency and was based on a conceptual model of nursing. Neither faculty knowledge nor the literature yielded a strategy for ensuring internal consistency and congruence. The literature between 1976 and 1980 contained little information related to the explication of the Neuman Systems Model and/or assistance in analyzing and evaluating the model for greater understanding of its use and its contribution to nursing education. The major resources for faculty from 1976 to 1980 were Neuman and Young (1972), "A Model for Teaching Total Person Approach to Patient Problems," and two chapters related to the Neuman Systems Model in Riehl and Roy (1974). Faculty drew heavily on publications related to systems theory by Selye (1950), von Bertalanffy (1968), Lazlo (1972), and Putt (1978), as well as works on curriculum development by authors such as Bevis (1978) and Torres and Yura (1974, 1975).

Betty Neuman became a primary resource and inspiration in 1980, after a telephone call to request approval of use of her graphic illustration of the Neuman Systems Model. Nursing faculty at Neumann College served as pioneers baccalaureate level in model implementation, and continue today to develop and improve the work as well as to consult with others who are interested in using the model in education, practice, and research. One of the members of the initial core group of faculty, Dr. Rosalie Mirenda, who developed the curriculum was selected by Dr. Neuman as the first president of the Neuman Systems Model Trustee Group, Inc., and continues to serve as a trustee today.

Associate Degree Program. The faculty at Neumann College who were implementing the model at the baccalaureate level served as experts for Cecil Community College. The faculty of both schools met on several occasions to compare definitions of terms, course content, care plan formats, and other curriculum documents. Eventually, the two programs developed an articulation model to facilitate student progression into a baccalaureate program.

Resources Needed

Baccalaureate Program. The need for resources that go beyond the critical but traditional financial support to operate a sound, accredited baccalaureate nursing program was implied throughout the experience of curriculum implementation by the Neumann College nursing program. A curriculum based on a clear and rational philosophy, learning theories, and the Neuman Systems Model as subject matter required the following resources or supports:

1. Leadership and commitment among the faculty to a value for conceptual models of nursing as central to the ongoing development of nursing knowledge and relevance to nursing education and practice.
2. Consensus among faculty to utilize a selected conceptual model of nursing as the subject matter for the curriculum.
3. Faculty with knowledge and understanding of the selected conceptual model of nursing and its implications for curriculum design.
4. Persistence, opportunities for faculty orientation, and ongoing education toward greater understanding of the selected conceptual model of nursing, the philosophy of curriculum, and the learning theory(ies), to ensure congruence among these components and an internally ordered curriculum.
5. Learners with characteristics facilitative of model use for learning nursing. In the case of the nursing curriculum based on the Neuman model, learners need a base knowledge of person as a wholistic being, systems, and integrated thinking.
6. Teaching–learning strategies facilitative of model integration and implementation. When using the Neuman model, the strategies need to actively engage the learner.
7. Teaching–learning settings that facilitate achievement of the purpose of nursing as set forth by the Neuman Systems Model: a need to accommodate client-centered and client-involved care planning and opportunity for delivering primary, secondary, and tertiary nursing prevention.
8. A process for curriculum review that improves and strengthens Neuman Systems Model implementation and eliminates constant curriculum revision unless motivated by new insights and understanding of the model's implications.

Documents describing the Neumann College nursing curriculum give evidence of the need for strong service leadership among the faculty in determining and providing the milieu for collaboration and team effort, and ensuring successful implementation and maintenance of the curriculum (Neumann College Division of Nursing, 1992).

Associate Degree Program.   Three members of the faculty were hired three months before the first class was to be admitted; their task was to develop the curriculum. The faculty and program director continued to meet once a month during the first year, to evaluate their progress as the curriculum was implemented. Between semesters, they also met for two- or three-day workshops to plan for the next semester. A curriculum consultant from the National League for Nursing (NLN) also provided guidance. Specific costs for the NLN consultation included $1,000 for two visits (1980 dollars) plus an additional $1,000 for room, board, and airfare—a total of $2,000. Additional costs for implementation included four faculty at full salary for three months of initial planning, and additional salary for all faculty as part of the team-building and clarification activities described earlier.

EXAMPLES OF IMPLEMENTATION

Assessment

Baccalaureate Program.   The achievement of optimum or maximum learning serves as the phenomenon of interest that relates to Neumann College nursing faculty's use of behavioristic, cognitive, and humanistic learning theories and related learning strategies. The faculty at Neumann College believe that teaching and learning are interrelated. They link learning to the learning activities and experiences designed to meet specific course objectives. Learning activities are constructed and sequenced with the intention of influencing the student's experience and thus the student's learning.

The multiple learning theories utilized by Neumann College's nursing faculty demonstrate consistency with a wholistic approach to the learner and learning and with the reciprocal interaction worldview. The nursing program is centered on the learner, who is viewed as an individual with unique learning needs and as an active participant in the learning process. Faculty believe that reciprocal interaction occurs between the learner and the learning environment and that change in behavior results from factors within the learner and the learning environment. Maximum learner achievement relates to the types of learning necessitated by the program subject matter, as guided by the Neuman Systems Model, and to the characteristics developed by the learner. Achievement is reflected in the program outcomes.

For assessment of the individual learner's degree of achievement of the objectives, input from faculty, students, and peers is sought. The collection of input from external sources—such as the National League for Nursing test scores and the National Council Licensure Examination (NCLEX), for assessment of the aggregate degree of achievement—allows evaluation of the effectiveness of the program.

Associate Degree Program.   Because this was a new program, the director determined a need to use a nursing model over the traditional medical model approach in curriculum development. Lowry used knowledge about nursing models from her doctoral study, in selecting the Neuman Systems Model for the curriculum at Cecil Community College. During the curriculum development process, the initial faculty conducted a thorough review of the literature and compared their philosophy and assumptions with those of the Neuman Systems Model to verify the appropriateness of the model's selection for the program (Lowry & Jopp, 1989). Consultants from Neumann College further aided in establishing the model's fit with the curriculum.

As noted earlier, the ease with which the language of the model is understood was a major advantage in implementing the model. The faculty expanded definitions of some variable concepts to include several subconcepts and also applied the model to the nursing education process itself. A model demonstrating the relationships among the client, student nurse, and faculty systems resulted (see Figure 5-2; Lowry, 1986; Lowry & Green, 1989).

Planning for Implementation of the Model

Enhancement and Inhibitions to Implementation—Baccalaureate Program.   The process of planning and implementing the curriculum based on the Neuman Systems Model at Neumann College followed a long and tedious course. The work related to the development of the curriculum was placed in the hands of small groups of faculty in ad hoc committees assigned by the director of the program. The faculty as a committee of the whole reviewed and approved recommendations from these ad hoc committees. The first task involved development of a document describing the conceptual framework, rationale, philosophy, purpose, objectives, and program outcomes. Once these were established, teams were organized to begin work on preprofessional learning and courses for the sophomore, junior, and senior levels. The faculty agreed that the curriculum committee, comprised of five faculty and the program director, would monitor the work. An ad hoc committee on the conceptual model, consisting of five members (two of whom were members of the curriculum committee), was charged to direct and accomplish the task of curriculum construction.

The five-member ad hoc committee began working on the task of curriculum development in September 1976, and met almost weekly for the first semester. Few resources were related to the development of a curriculum utilizing a conceptual model of nursing as its guiding framework. The faculty did not select a specific curriculum development model or process. However, the faculty's perspective on components of curriculum appeared to be consistent with Beauchamp's (1972) view of curriculum, which emphasizes philosophy, subject matter, and learning theory as essential components. Bevis (1973, 1982) and Torres and Yura (1974, 1975) served as major references during the process of curriculum development. The group struggled with understanding and interpreting the few available primary and secondary sources related to the use of conceptual models of nursing. A member of the faculty planning group described the struggle:

> *The visibility of the concepts of the Neuman model in curriculum and the ownership by total faculty—those there at the time and those to join us in the future—were the priorities. These were difficult days, filled with debate, compromise, battles of semantics, meetings, long days and even longer sets of minutes and reports. Literature searches resulted in disappointment for the most part. The struggle continued and, slowly, but surely, faculty began to take some risk and statement of objectives, course syllabi and assessment tools emerged. Throughout it all, optimism remained within a core group of faculty. It was right to seek a way in which*

the medical model could be subsumed in its rightful place within the nursing curriculum, that is, within the context of a wholistic nursing approach, utilizing the Neuman Systems Model. (Mirenda, 1986b, p. 2.3)

Enhancement and Inhibitions to Implementation—Associate Degree Program.   The development of a new associate degree program at Cecil Community College proved to be beneficial in that no adaptations of an existing curriculum were required. Selection of the model by Lowry prior to hiring any of the faculty also allowed potential faculty members to better determine their compatibility with the program. Despite this advantage, some faculty with previous teaching experience exhibited resistance to change. The result was inconsistency in the manner in which the model was implemented throughout the curriculum. The resistance necessitated intervention to clarify the problems and establish a constant and congruous approach. The availability of resources for consultation, networking, and employment of faculty, without teaching responsibilities, for three months prior to implementation enabled a more thorough understanding and internalization of the model and resulted in greater consistency in its use.

Consistency with Mission and Proposed Use of Model.   All undergraduate nursing education programs seek to provide students with knowledge to guide their practice, and faculty attempt to impart the information in a manner that facilitates retention and application. Use of nursing models affords an organized structure for mastery or nursing knowledge, and the Neuman Systems Model adapts readily to associate and baccalaureate education.

Nursing faculty at Neumann College believe that incorporating a specific conceptual model of nursing (i.e., the Neuman Systems Model) as an essential component for curriculum construction proposes a theoretical perspective in nursing. A model identifies and emphasizes concepts, theories, and process essential to the understanding and practice of professional nursing. Utilization of the Neuman Systems Model for curriculum construction (a) enhances the potential for distinguishing professional from technical practice while meeting the teaching–learning needs of those who select professional nursing practice; (b) facilitates a teaching–learning environment that values theory and fosters theoretical identity in future practitioners of nursing; and (c) promotes the development of the science of nursing by focusing the research process on phenomena significant to nursing, rather than an atheoretical research skill/process acquisition mode.

If nursing aspires to influence practice and health care delivery systems through application and testing of nursing theory, content related to the purpose, generation, and use of theory must be part of curriculum design. Not only must nursing students be conversant with theory before entering doctoral programs, but first-level practitioners also require knowledge and ability in the use of theory as well as an appreciation for its value (Jacobs-Kramer & Huether, 1988). Beginning professional (baccalaureate) students must be introduced to the rationale and techniques in theory-based practice as well as to the history of nursing knowledge, conceptual models for nursing practice, research, education, and tools and techniques for using and judging their adequacy. Neumann College nursing faculty assist baccalaureate students in developing an ability to deal with theory so as to begin to appreciate the necessity for theory and their participation in the further development of nursing knowledge, a long-recognized component of the profession (Meleis & Price, 1988).

The mission of associate degree education in nursing includes two other areas that support the use of the Neuman Systems Model in nursing curricula. First, associate degree education prepares direct caregivers primarily for institutional settings. The model's use of primary, secondary, and tertiary prevention as intervention allows educators to focus intervention on role-appropriate activities in a progressive manner. Second, associate degree education establishes a foundation for baccalaureate-level education. Use of the Neuman Systems Model could provide a common knowledge base to facilitate continuation in nursing education (Lowry, 1986).

Tasks to Be Performed in Implementation

The work of implementation of a conceptual model of nursing in curriculum requires understanding of the potential contributions of the nursing model, the faculty's philosophy of curriculum, and learning theories to a logically congruent curriculum. Strong external and internal pressures, such as changes in health care environment, changes in characteristics of students entering nursing programs, faculty's strong individual interests, and competitive markets, force nursing educators to make decisions affecting curriculum (Conrad & Pratt, 1983). These decisions, however, often result in the addition of new content, new strategies, and new clinical experiences rather than purposeful actions based on an organized strategy that achieves compatibility among its components and is directed at agreed-on educational aims. Fawcett's (1995) framework for analysis and evaluation of conceptual models of nursing, and Mirenda's (1995) strategy for analysis and evaluation of essential components of curriculum complement one another and provide the nursing faculty with tools to link a conceptual model of nursing with their philosophy and theories about teaching–learning for coherent curriculum construction.

Program Heads.   A number of strategies mentioned earlier for successful implementation of the Neuman Systems Model should be incorporated into the strategic planning by program directors. Lowry and Jopp (1989) noted the importance of creation of an environment conducive to communication, collaboration, and creativity in a relaxed setting. Program heads need to establish a specific schedule for implementation, with long- and short-term goals clearly delineated. They also should define the roles of the individuals involved and assist faculty in developing network relationships with other programs that have successfully implemented the model.

Faculty.   Faculty need to focus on reviewing materials about the model and establishing definitions for concepts. They also need to determine the scope of the model within the program. Faculty may find it helpful to keep notebooks on ideas related to implementation of the model.

Impact of Target Audience on Implementation of the Model

Nursing practice as described by Neuman (1982, 1989, 1995) requires the development and refinement of mental processes that are consistent with the outcomes desired and that include reflective and rational, syntactical, contextual, and inquiry learning. Reflective and rational learning uses theory to inform practice. Syntactical learning sees meaningful wholes, relationships, and patterns; provides individualized, unique client care; gains insights; and collaboratively finds meaning in client system response. Contextual learning develops a multidimensional and context-dependent view of reality. Inquiry learning encompasses creativity, investigation, theorizing, identifying, clarifying, and predicting.

Neuman's ideas about nurses and nursing practice seem congruent with contemporary education thought:

> *Teachers create the climate of the course—its contextual reality. It is they who determine whether the learner will be active or passive, whether their realities will be context free or context based, and whether they will view wholes or parts. Learning has degrees between passive and active. (Bevis, 1989, p. 222)*

Bevis goes on to say that active learning requires knowledge to be dissected, analyzed, rearranged, and examined for underlying assumptions; used to project implications; compared with other known data; and made part of the system of knowledge owned by the learner.

The Neumann College nursing program faculty identified, early in the program's history, the need for active faculty–learner participation as well as integrated and wholistic approaches to the understanding of person and to nursing practice. These basic beliefs about types of learning coincide with the character of nursing practice delineated by the Neuman Systems Model and reinforced by contemporary thought in nursing education.

In nursing education, faculty, students, and clients, who comprise the target audience, possess diverse educational preparation and skills levels. Faculty generally possess graduate degrees in nursing, practice in the clinical setting, and some experience with nursing models. They either respond enthusiastically to implementation of the model, or they resist change from existing practice. Communication plays a key role in ensuring consistency in interpretation of the model (Lowry & Jopp, 1989).

Students usually are novices in knowledge regarding nursing models and clinical skills. A general introduction to the entire model, followed by progressive implementation of it, seems to work best with students. The educational and experience background of nontraditional students may impact their reception of the model. For example, licensed practical nurses or registered nurses who have returned to school to advance their nursing education may experience greater difficulty in accepting the model if it deviates significantly from their previous educational approach.

Clients typically have no experience with nursing models and possess varying levels of health care knowledge. Among the nursing models, the Neuman Systems Model works well with the lay population, which comprises the majority of clients in the health care system. The use of common terms increases their comfort with the model, and the wholistic approach, which involves the client in health care decisions, fits in well with today's more informed health care consumers.

SUPPORT NEEDED FOR IMPLEMENTATION

Successful implementation relies on effective leadership, commitment to theory-based nursing, and adequate funding. As discussed earlier, the individual responsible for assisting faculty in implementing the model must provide leadership throughout the curriculum process. Difficulties may arise, and maintenance of strong communication will prove critical. The change also requires an intensive investment of time and effort, and fiscal resources must be present to allow for the creative component of curriculum development and to provide opportunities for consultation and networking (Lowry & Jopp, 1989).

The existence of a value for the theoretical identity of future practitioners of nursing, and a philosophy and learning theories that are congruent with the specific model of nursing selected, serve as the major support for construction and implementation of a curriculum based on a conceptual model of nursing. At Neumann College, the nursing program faculty articulated a sound belief in systems thinking and in the importance of theoretical foundations to conceptualization and to the preparation of professional nurses. The Neuman Systems Model is based on general systems theory. Its concepts and propositions constitute the conceptual basis of the baccalaureate curriculum. Through the conceptual model (and the theoretical perspective of systems from which it is derived), the nursing faculty provides a broad theoretical foundation that will enable the professional nurse to practice competently, examine and critique practice, hypothesize about the nature of nursing, and, eventually, contribute to theory that further defines the discipline of nursing and nursing practice.

APPLICATION OF PRINCIPLES OF STRATEGIC PLANNING

Specific Objectives to Be Achieved in Implementation of the Model

Goals established as a result of discussion and analysis of the external and internal forces that were potential or actual for Neumann College's nursing program included curriculum construction, implementation, and evaluation of the process and of the resultant curriculum. External forces—advances in computerization, changes in professional accreditation criteria, and demographic shifts creating a high potential for diversity in future student populations—affected the context for curriculum development utilizing the Neuman Systems Model, but the major forces influencing the revision emanated from within the institution and the nursing program.

As a basis for strategic planning and goal setting, the college faculty revisited and reaffirmed the philosophy and mission, and continued to voice commitment to the value of the liberal arts in the preparation for profession. Concurrently, leading nurse scholars and authors had explicated a metaparadigm distinct from those of other health professions (Donaldson & Crowley, 1978; Fawcett, 1984). Neumann College's nursing faculty accepted this emerging metaparadigm as foundational to any future discussion of the discipline of nursing. Thus began the journey to curriculum development with the Neuman Systems Model as the subject matter/discipline.

The objectives for implementation of the model at Cecil Community College included establishing a curriculum based on a nursing model, providing students with a means for organizing their knowledge base, and providing graduates with a model on which to base their practice for a changing health care system.

Timeline

The work of developing, maintaining, and evaluating the Neuman-based nursing curriculum at Neumann College began in 1974 and continues today. Initial curriculum development and implementation occurred between 1976 and 1984. The curriculum received state board approval in March 1979, and the program has undergone two reaccreditation visits by the National League for Nursing in 1984 and 1992. In both instances, the program received full eight-year approval with no recommendations for curriculum. Results from the program's comprehensive evaluation system for each specific year are included in the program's annual report. The years since 1984 reflect ongoing evaluation and modification, but no *major* revision.

Cecil Community College implemented the model over a two-year period. Faculty defined terms, mapped out the curriculum, and developed the first-year courses during the first three months. Client care plans and clinical evaluation tools were developed as the program progressed. During the first year of the curriculum, monthly meetings were scheduled to monitor progress. Between the fall and spring semesters, the faculty spent two or three days meeting to finalize plans for the following semester. The second year followed a similar pattern: three months were spent in developing the second-year courses and the implementation occurred during the academic year. Lowry and Jopp (1989) also developed the instrument described in the "Evaluation" section, which appears later in the chapter, to evaluate internalization and use of the Neuman Systems Model by graduates.

Task Assignment

At Cecil Community College, the entire faculty worked together in writing the philosophy, objectives (both terminal and level), and glossary. Then they divided into pairs (according to specialty areas) to develop courses. Efforts were made to accommodate special interests in making assignments.

TIPS FOR SUCCESS

Concrete Tips

The experience of the curriculum development and implementation process at Neumann College suggests that three major factors need to exist for long-term success, defined as continuation of a Neuman-based curriculum over time:

1. A conceptual model, such as the Neuman Systems Model, that is comprehensive and detailed enough to provide answers and details for curriculum design—a conceptual model that responds to Fawcett's (1995) rules for education.
2. A faculty that has knowledge of the conceptual model and a commitment to and value for (a) theoretical identity in future practitioners in nursing and (b) a logically congruent curriculum based on a conceptual model of nursing as a means for developing theoretical perspectives in nursing.
3. Leadership that is creative, energetic, and facilitative of a decision-making process that provides opportunity for participation by all nursing faculty and opportunity for nonnurse faculty in the college to have input into the final curriculum design. (Other success factors to consider were addressed earlier in this chapter.)

Several other tips for successful implementation of the model were outlined by Lowry and Jopp (1989). Table 5-1 includes 15 of those strategies.

Methods to Ensure Model Integrity

Baccalaureate Program.   At Neumann College, the emphasis on curriculum integrity revolves around an orientation to, and ongoing continuing education (formal and informal) on, matters of

Table 5–1
Strategies for Successful Implementation of the
Neuman Systems Model

1. Review the literature about the model.
2. Define the constructs of the model.
3. Define the scope of the model for the intended program.
4. Encourage faculty to choose areas of exploration and development in which they are most interested.
5. Share agreeably the responsibilities among the members.
6. Provide opportunities for team building and values clarification.
7. Set specific times for faculty work sessions.
8. Select locations conducive to productivity and free from interruptions.
9. Maintain an informal atmosphere at work sessions.
10. Encourage creativity, risk taking, and innovation.
11. Eliminate "tunnel vision" and criticism.
12. Establish a written timetable for short- and long-term goals.
13. Appoint one member to keep group interaction notes, and review them from session to session to provide continuity.
14. Encourage members to keep idea logs in which they record creative thoughts, strategies, and ideas.
15. Establish a network with faculties from other institutions that utilize the model.

"An Evaluation Instrument for Assessing an Associate Degree Nursing Curriculum Based on the Neuman Systems Model" by L. W. Lowry and M. C. Jopp, 1989. In J. Riehl-Sisca (Ed.), *Conceptual Models for Nursing Practice* (3rd ed., p. 76). Norwalk, CT: Appleton & Lange. Used with permission.

curriculum, the Neuman Systems Model, and its implementation. A curriculum committee oversees the curriculum evaluation and revision process, thus monitoring the ongoing appropriate use of the model in course development and clinical application. Model integrity is viewed as an ethical consideration by faculty who value and engage in scholarly activity. Faculty are expected to maintain and develop their knowledge of the Neuman Systems Model and to participate in research activity as it relates to use of the model for the curriculum and the character of the practice learned by the students.

Associate Degree Program. At Cecil Community College, the faculty was small (four in first year; seven in second year), and they monitored each other. Frequent meetings were scheduled over lunch and in each other's homes, combining work with social time.

The faculty liked and trusted each other and worked together with no hidden agendas. As years went on and new faculty joined the ranks, those from the original team committed to orient and mentor new faculty in order to maintain integrity in course development and implementation according to the model.

EVALUATION

Evaluation Processes for Implementation

Baccalaureate Program. The Neumann College nursing program faculty ensure a logical and consistent curriculum based on the Neuman Systems Model through an oversight curriculum committee, content mapping, course faculty-student teams, and a systematic plan for evaluation. The faculty intends that these processes assist faculty's knowledge of the subject matter to be learned and of the content that is foundational to the learning of the discipline. The characteristics of the students are assessed and assisted through the admission process and the liberal arts preparation that undergirds the learning of the discipline of nursing as delineated by the Neuman Systems Model.

Learning theories and teaching-learning methods selected have optimal or maximum learning as the desired outcome. Annual reports indicate that the nursing program's average attrition rate of 10% ranks below the national average. Employment rates in the field for the nursing graduate continue to average 97%. One might infer from such statistics that the curriculum and its related teaching-learning strategies assist the learners to successfully complete the nursing program and find employment. A direct cause-effect relationship, however, cannot be inferred (Mirenda, 1995).

A graduate follow-up study, conducted every three years, contains questions related to the graduates' continued use of the major Neuman model concepts and propositions in their practice. Results to date indicate graduates' continued integration of the concepts of wholism, interdependent client system variables, and three levels of prevention as interventions (Neumann College Division of Nursing, 1992).

Associate Degree Program.   The evaluation process for the associate degree program at Cecil Community College was conceived during the planning phase for the program. The guidelines provided by the NLN gave direction for the areas of evaluation needed throughout the two-year program. Client care plans and clinical evaluation tools reflected the concepts in the model and were leveled to accommodate student progression through the program. These methods of formative evaluations represented universal approaches for educational programs. The unique evaluative process for this program consisted of the development of an instrument to assess graduates' internalization and use of the model to guide practice. The instrument was developed in three steps: (a) selecting the constructs to be measured, (b) formulating the test items, and (c) testing the instrument for reliability and validity (Lowry & Jopp, 1989). The final instrument contained 90 items: 44 in the first section, which measured internalization of the model, and 46 in the second section, which measured use of the model in practice. The instrument was completed by seniors three weeks before graduation and then eight months after graduation. Five classes participated in the longitudinal study from 1985 through 1989. Findings revealed that graduates internalized the constructs well, and no change occurred over time. However, the use of the model in practice showed great variation. In settings where knowledge of the model existed and supervisors supported model-based practice, graduates demonstrated greater use of the model to guide practice. On the other hand, graduates receiving no support in the use of the model failed to use it (Lowry, 1995).

The Lowry-Jopp Neuman Model Evaluation Instrument (LJNMEI) was refined by the faculty at Indiana University–Purdue University at Fort Wayne, and the new edition is currently being used to assess their graduates' use and internalization of the model. The faculty at Cecil Community College believe that model-based programs must be evaluated to test their efficacy. Today, the trend is moving away from models to guide curriculum. The National League for Nursing no longer mandates the use of models. Those who believe in the efficacy of models to guide curriculum, practice, and research are concerned by the elimination of models. Organizing frameworks have proven to be successful in businesses, companies, hospitals, and myriad other organizations composed of large numbers of people, data, and subdivisions. Nursing models serve a similar organizational purpose. Nurses educated from a model-based program possess an advantage over their colleagues. Not only are they equipped to practice wholistic care, but, as they progress to higher levels of nursing education, they can transfer the knowledge they possess about one framework to others. Knowledge built on a good foundation need not be discarded to relearn new ways. Providing a firm foundation serves as the key to continuous successful learning. Program evaluation represents a vital force in facilitating responsible nursing education.

OTHER EXAMPLES OF USE OF THE NEUMAN SYSTEMS MODEL

The use of the Neuman Systems Model in nursing education is described in both publications and presentations (Bourbonnais & Ross, 1985; Kilchenstein & Yakulis, 1984; Leobold & Davis, 1980; Lowry, 1986; Marriner, 1986; Mirenda, 1986). More specifically, Bower (1982) has identified a blueprint consistent with the Neuman Systems Model that gives direction for the generation of the overall program and level outcomes of the curriculum, the content and its sequence, and the course descriptions. Bower emphasizes that each step of the curriculum development process depends on creating internal consistency between the original conceptual model selected and the final course construction. Knox, Kilchenstein, and Yakulis (1982) provided a description of a four-year integrated program based on an adaptation of the Neuman Systems Model and designed to provide a wholistic curriculum focused on care of individuals, families, and communities.

A paper presented by Neuman in 1985 identified a list of schools in the United States, Canada, and abroad, that utilize the Neuman Systems Model. The second edition of the Neuman Systems Model text, edited by Betty Neuman in 1989, contained an entire section describing the application of the Neuman Systems Model to nursing education. Examples of the application of the Neuman model include baccalaureate and graduate nursing programs at California

State University, Fresno (Stittich, Avent, & Patterson, 1989), a cooperative baccalaureate education program in Minnesota (Mrkonich, Hessian, & Miller, 1989), a baccalaureate North Dakota–Minnesota nursing education consortium (Nelson, Hansen, & McCullagh, 1989), an associate degree program in transition to a baccalaureate program (Sipple & Freese, 1989), a baccalaureate program undergoing curriculum revision at the University of Saskatchewan (Dyck, Innes, Rae, & Sawatzky, 1989), and utilization of the Neuman model in multilevel nurse education programs at the University of Nevada (Louis, Witt, & LaMancusa, 1989).

The University of Tennessee at Martin also based a curriculum of its BSN program on the Neuman Systems Model when the program was established in 1989 to replace an associate degree program. As part of the curriculum development process, the faculty converted existing associate degree-level clinical evaluation tools to baccalaureate-level tools based on the Neuman Systems Model and using the model's terminology. The tools use four rating classifications and define specific behaviors in each of the four ratings for the 25 items included in the clinical evaluation. Emphasis on the model concepts progresses through each of the program's three levels, and the tools reflect the leveling approach (Seng, 1995).

The Neuman Systems Model's ready implementation in education will ensure its popularity. The number of nursing education programs adopting the model is expected to continue to grow.

REFERENCES

Beauchamp, G. (1972). Basic components of a curriculum theory. *Curriculum Theory Network, 10,* 16–22.

Bevis, E. M. (1973). *Curriculum building in nursing: A process.* New York: National League for Nursing.

Bevis, E. M. (1978). *Curriculum building in nursing: A process.* New York: National League for Nursing.

Bevis, E. M. (1982). *Curriculum building in nursing: A process.* New York: National League for Nursing.

Bevis, E. M. (1989). *Curriculum building in nursing: A process.* New York: National League for Nursing.

Bourbonnais, F., & Ross, M. (1985). The Neuman Systems Model in nursing education: Course development and implementation. *Journal of Advanced Nursing, 10,* 117-123.

Bower, F. L. (1982). Curriculum development and the Neuman model. In B. Neuman, *The Neuman Systems Model: Application to nursing education and practice* (pp. 94-99). Norwalk, CT: Appleton-Century-Crofts.

Caplan, G. (1964). *Principles of preventive psychiatry.* New York: Basic Books.

Conrad, C. F., & Pratt, A. M. (1983). Making decisions about the curriculum. *Journal of Higher Education, 54,* 16-30.

Cornu, A. (1957). *The origins of Marxist thought.* Springfield, IL: Thomas.

Donaldson, S. K., & Crowley, D. M. (1978). The discipline of nursing. *Nursing Outlook, 16,* 113-120.

Donley, Sr. R. (1989). Curriculum revolution: Heeding the voices of change. In *Curriculum revolution: Reconceptualizing nursing education* (pp. 1-8). New York: National League for Nursing.

Dyck, S. M., Innes, J. E., Rae, D. I., & Sawatzky, J. E. (1989). The Neuman Systems Model in curriculum revision: A baccalaureate program, University of Saskatchewan. In B. Neuman (Ed.), *The Neuman Systems Model* (2nd ed., pp. 225-236). Norwalk, CT: Appleton & Lange.

Edelson, M. (1970). *Sociotherapy and psychotherapy.* Chicago: University of Chicago Press.

Emery, F. (Ed.). (1969). *Systems thinking.* Baltimore: Penguin Books.

Fawcett, J. (1984). The metaparadigm of nursing: Current status and future refinements. *Image: The Journal of Nursing Scholarship, 16,* 84-87.

Fawcett, J. (1989). *Analysis and evaluation of conceptual models of nursing* (2nd ed.). Philadelphia: Davis.

Fawcett, J. (1995). *Analysis and evaluation of conceptual models of nursing* (3rd ed.). Philadelphia: Davis.

Jacobs-Kramer, M. K., & Huether, S. E. (1988). Curricular considerations for teaching nursing theory. *Journal of Professional Nursing, 4,* 373-380.

Kilchenstein, L., & Yakulis, I. (1984). The birth of a curriculum: Utilization of the Betty Neuman health-care systems model. *Journal of Nursing Education, 23,* 126-127.

Knox, J. E., Kilchenstein, L., & Yakulis, I. M. (1982). Utilization of the Neuman model in an integrated baccalaureate program: University of Pittsburgh. In B. Neuman (Ed.), *The Neuman Systems Model* (2nd ed., pp. 117-123). Norwalk, CT: Appleton & Lange.

Lazlo, E. (1972). *The systems view of the world: The natural philosophy of the new development in the sciences.* New York: Braziller.

Leobold, M., & Davis, L. (1980). A baccalaureate nursing curriculum based on the Neuman health systems model. In J. P. Riehl & C. Roy (Eds.), *Conceptual models for nursing practice* (2nd ed., pp. 151–158). New York: Appleton-Century-Crofts.

Louis, M., Witt, R., & LaMancusa, M. (1989). The Neuman Systems Model in multilevel nurse education programs: University of Nevada, Las Vegas. In B. Neuman (Ed.), *The Neuman Systems Model* (2nd ed., pp. 237–248). Norwalk, CT: Appleton & Lange.

Lowry, L. (1986). Adapted by degrees. *Senior Nurse, 5*(3), 10–12.

Lowry, L. W. (1995). *Efficacy of the Neuman Systems Model as a curriculum framework: A longitudinal study.* Manuscript submitted for publication.

Lowry, L. W., & Green, G. H. (1989). Four Neuman-based associate degree nursing programs: Brief description and evaluation. In B. Neuman (Ed.), *The Neuman Systems Model: Application to nursing education and practice* (2nd ed., pp. 283–312). Norwalk, CT: Appleton & Lange.

Lowry, L. W., & Jopp, M. C. (1989). An evaluation instrument for assessing an associate degree nursing curriculum based on the Neuman Systems Model. In J. Riehl-Sisca (Ed.), *Conceptual models for nursing practice* (3rd ed., pp. 73–85). Norwalk, CT: Appleton & Lange.

Marriner, A. (1986). *Nursing theorists and their work.* St. Louis: Mosby.

Meleis, A. I., & Price, M. (1988). Strategies and conditions for teaching theoretical nursing: An international perspective. *Journal of Advanced Nursing, 3,* 592–604.

Mirenda, R. M. (1986a). The Neuman Systems Model: Description and application. In P. Winstead-Fry (Ed.), *Case studies in nursing theory* (pp. 127–166). New York: National League for Nursing.

Mirenda, R. M. (1986b). The Neuman Systems Model and nursing education for a new age: A ten-year journey. *Proceedings of the First International Symposium on the Neuman Systems Model* (pp. 2.1–2.6). Aston, PA: Neumann College.

Mirenda, R. M. (1995). *A conceptual-theoretical strategy for curriculum development in baccalaureate nursing programs.* Unpublished doctoral dissertation, Widener University, Chester, PA.

Mrkonich, D. E., Hessian, M., & Miller, M. W. (1989). A cooperative process in curriculum development using the Neuman health-care systems model. In J. P. Riehl-Sisca, *Conceptual models for nursing practice* (3rd ed., pp. 87–94). Norwalk, CT: Appleton & Lange.

Nelson, L., Hansen, M., & McCullagh, M. (1989). A new baccalaureate North Dakota–Minnesota nursing education consortium. In B. Neuman (Ed.), *The Neuman Systems Model* (2nd ed., pp. 183–192). Norwalk, CT: Appleton & Lange.

Neuman, B. (1980). The Betty Neuman health-care systems model: A total person approach to patient problems. In J. P. Riehl & C. Roy, *Conceptual models for nursing practice* (2nd ed., pp. 119–134). New York: Appleton-Century-Crofts.

Neuman, B. (1982a). The Neuman health-care systems model: A total approach to client care. In B. Neuman (Ed.), *The Neuman Systems Model: Application to nursing education and practice* (pp. 8–29). Norwalk, CT: Appleton-Century-Crofts.

Neuman, B. (1982b). The systems concept and nursing. In B. Neuman (Ed.), *The Neuman Systems Model: Application to nursing education and practice* (pp. 3–7). Norwalk, CT: Appleton-Century-Crofts.

Neuman, B. (1985, August). *The Neuman Systems Model.* Paper presented at the Nursing Theory in Action Conference, Edmonton, Canada.

Neuman, B. (1989). The Neuman Systems Model. In B. Neuman (Ed.), *The Neuman Systems Model: Application to nursing education and practice* (2nd ed., pp. 3–63). Norwalk, CT: Appleton & Lange.

Neuman, B. (1995). The Neuman Systems Model. In B. Neuman (Ed.), *The Neuman Systems Model: Application to nursing education and practice* (3rd ed., pp. 3–61). Norwalk, CT: Appleton & Lange.

Neuman, B., & Young, R. J. (1972). A model for teaching total person approach to patient problems. *Nursing Research, 21,* 264–269.

Neumann College Nursing Program. (1984). *Self evaluation report based on the National League for Nursing criteria for the approval of baccalaureate and higher degree programs in nursing* (Vol. 1). Aston, PA: Author.

Neumann College Division of Nursing. (1992). *Self-study report based on the National League for Nursing guidelines for preparation for reaccreditation* (Vol. 1). Aston, PA: Author.

Putt, A. M. (1978). *General systems theory applied to nursing.* Boston: Little, Brown.

Riehl, J. P., & Roy, C. (1974). *Conceptual models for nursing practice.* New York: Appleton-Century-Crofts.

Scales, F. (1985). *Nursing curriculum: Development, structure, function.* Norwalk, CT: Appleton-Century-Crofts.

Selye, H. (1950). *Physiology and pathology of exposure to stress.* Montreal, Canada: ACTA.

Seng, V. S. (1995). The Neuman Systems Model in clinical evaluation of students. In B. Neuman (Ed.), *The Neuman Systems Model: Application to nursing education and practice* (3rd ed., pp. 215–225). Norwalk, CT: Appleton & Lange.

Sipple, J. A., & Freese, B. T. (1989). Transition from technical to professional-level nursing education. In B. Neuman (Ed.), *The Neuman Systems Model* (2nd ed., pp. 193–200). Norwalk, CT: Appleton & Lange.

Stittich, E. M., Avent, C. L., & Patterson, K. (1989). Neuman based baccalaureate and graduate nursing programs, California State University, Fresno. In B. Neuman (Ed.), *The Neuman Systems Model* (2nd ed., pp. 163–174). Norwalk, CT: Appleton & Lange.

Teilhard de Chardin, P. (1955). *The phenomenon of man.* London: Collins.

Torres, G., & Yura, H. (1974). *Today's conceptual framework: Its relationship to the curriculum development process.* New York: National League for Nursing.

Torres, G., & Yura, H. (1975). The conceptual framework as part of the curriculum process. In *Conceptual framework—Its meaning and function* (pp. 41–53). New York: National League for Nursing.

von Bertalanffy, L. (1968). *General system theory.* New York: Braziller.

An updated complete list of categorized Neuman-based citations has been compiled by Dr. J. Fawcett at the end of the *Neuman Systems Model,* third edition (1995). Norwalk, CT: Appleton & Lang.

The 1995 Neuman text also included Neuman Trustee names and addresses (22 members) who offer support in understanding and implementing the Neuman Systems Model worldwide.

Major Concepts Represented in the Neuman Systems Model, and the Philosophical Claims of the Neumann College Nursing Program Faculty

Major Concept	Neuman Systems Model, Neumann College Nursing Program (1984)	Neumann College Nursing Faculty (Mirenda, 1995)
Person–Environment	Client systems are open systems that interact with the environment in order to promote harmony and balance between the internal and external environments. Environment involves both internal and external stressors.	Client systems are open, living systems with interdependent parts in interaction with the environment. Client systems interact with stressors in the environment that are intra-, extra-, and interpersonal.
Learner	See Person-Environment (above)	This curriculum enhances students' knowledge of their own and others' interdependent spiritual, sociocultural, physical, and psychologic components.
Learner–Environment	See Person-Environment (above)	Learning takes place best in an academic atmosphere that facilitates faculty-student interaction.
Health	Represents a usual dynamic stability state of the normal line of defense. Client systems' position on their wellness–illness continuum is related to the amount of available energy.	Wholistic, encompassing the five variables of the client system. It is the ability of the system to function at the optimal level of its capabilities, to respond effectively to stress.
Students' Learning	See Health (above)	Students are encouraged to view themselves as developing professional nurses who are responsible for determining their learning, with faculty input as needed.

Major Concept	Neuman Systems Model, Neumann College Nursing Program (1984)	Neumann College Nursing Faculty (Mirenda, 1995)
Nursing	Concerned with reduction of potential or actual stressor reaction through use of primary, secondary, and tertiary preventions as interventions to retain, attain, and maintain system stability or wellness. Perceptual distortions between client and nurse are mutually negotiated and resolved.	A professional service; the expression of the dedicated person, utilizing scholarly/scientific principles. It is a dynamic, preventive, therapeutic, rehabilitative service that assists client systems to retain, attain, and maintain an optimal level of well-being.
Education	See Nursing (above)	Learners' total development is reinforced and extended to others through a strong liberal arts and professional program. Faculty and students evaluate the experience available for successful development. The design of the academic programs, with their choices, reflects the climate of freedom in which the faculty seeks to assist the learner in the search for learning and continued development in making responsible choices.

6

Watson's Theory of Transpersonal Caring

M. Jean Watson

*T*his chapter offers a blueprint for Watson's theory of human caring, also referred to as transpersonal caring. This work, begun in 1979 and continually developed until this moment in history, is described herein. The early theory books for this work are: *Nursing: The Philosophy and Science of Caring* (1979/1985) and *Nursing: Human Science and Human Care* (1985/1988c). This chapter also integrates some of the author's latest thinking, based on other publications and on a major, comprehensive text in progress.

The scope of this work focuses primarily on the centrality of human caring and on the caring-to-caring transpersonal relationship and its healing potential for both the one who is caring and the one who is being cared for. The original work (1979/1985) offered a structure and order for nursing's "core components" as a "basis for understanding and studying the basic foundation of nursing" (p. xx). The "core" was conceptualized around ten carative factors that are basic to nursing and which are discussed more explicitly later in this chapter.

The evolving work-in-progress is geared toward a paradigmatic structure for the whole of nursing and its emergence as a distinct caring-healing-health discipline and profession for the next century.

Although the broad disciplinary and professional context will be referenced in this "blueprint," the focus for this chapter will be on the original "theory" and its most contemporary evolving components, not the current work-in-progress, which is related to the caring-healing paradigmatic matrix. This later work will be published elsewhere as a free-standing book.

To enter into these ideas, it should first be noted that the concepts need continual study, development, and research. They may help to guide the study of nursing, and the emergence of its art and science of caring knowledge and practices, because the focus has implications for health and healing practices and processes. It is thus acknowledged that nursing is both scientific and artistic; it exists as a human science discipline as well as an academic-clinical profession. Its professional ethic resides in a human relational-human service calling. Nursing's caring-healing knowledge and practices are drawn from the arts and humanities as well as from traditional and emerging sciences.

Because caring and human caring-healing relations are considered central and foundational to the whole of nursing (theory, practice, education, research, and administration), it is somewhat impossible to focus here on any one of these from an "application" point of view; in other words, my caring work is considered, and can be read as: *a philosophy, an ethic, a conceptual model, or a specific theory.* At this point in its evolution, I consider my most current work "beyond theory"—it is more a philosophical, ethical, intellectual blueprint for nursing's evolving disciplinary/professional matrix. Nevertheless, others interact with the original work at multiple levels of concreteness or abstractness, and it has been and is being "applied" in education, practice, research, and administration in nursing and, in some instances, in other fields.

I want to point out that this work is offered as a nonprescriptive model, an invitation for nursing and nurses to consider these ideas in the loose-definition sense of theory. Consider the Greek word *theorēma,* that is, using this work as a guide to see, "to keep one's gaze fixed upon," some truths about the ground of nursing's being and becoming (paradoxically, both as it currently is, but is not; and also what it might become yet ironically is already becoming). In a sense, these values, ideas, and ethics of caring and healing are already dormant, latent, and inscribed in nursing's evolving history.

In working with any nursing theory or nursing model at many levels, the real success lies in the reflective nature of the process nurses engage in; further, it is important for all engaged in such activities to adopt a critical stance whereby the values and beliefs of the theory work together. One is not detached from the other; each informs the other. Ultimately, practice evolves toward "praxis," closing the theory–practice gap between the "caring ideal" and what an informed, reflective, caring nurse actually does. How the nurse experiences caring as ontology merges with her or his actions.

It is important to heed the advice and insight of Pearson (1983) and Johns (1994) in their work on the Burford Nursing Development Unit Project in Oxford, England. I quote Pearson:

> *No model can be accepted as final representation of reality, but only as a basis for further analysis, concept identification, theory building, and testing leading to a dynamic and developing approach to the practice of nursing. (p. 55)*

However, because this work posits a value's explicit philosophical and moral foundation, and because this "theory" takes a specific position with respect to the centrality of human caring as an ethic, an ontology, and a critical starting point for nursing's *raison d'être,* it can be used as a guide to any aspect of nursing and health care. Nevertheless, it is dependent on critical, reflective practices that must be continuously questioned and critiqued in order to remain dynamic, flexible, and endlessly self-revising and evolving.

Background

The concepts for some aspects of this work were derived from clinically inducted experiences, combined with my philosophical, intellectual, and experiential background. The theory emerged from my own values, beliefs, and perceptions about human life, health, and healing, which were manifest clinically and empirically in my experiences and observations. I saw nursing's collective caring-healing role and its mission in society as attending to, and helping to sustain, humanity and wholeness. To me, these were foundational to nursing's purpose.

My original work (1979/1985) was also influenced by phenomenological psychology and philosophy; for example, the phenomenological psychology of Carl Rogers, the existential work of Yalom, and the interpersonal focus gained from psychiatric-mental health nursing studies and Peplau's interpersonal domain. Other intellectual influences included the philosophies of Kierkegaard, Whitehead, Teilhard de Chardin, and Sartre. Another early intellectual influence was the work of Richard Lazarus and his use of the term *transpersonal* with respect to the human stress-coping experience. This term later found support and congruence and further explicit development in the formal branch of transpersonal psychology. My more recent, evolving work on transpersonal caring is closely related to the concepts in transpersonal psychology, although my original derivation of the term from Lazarus has been modified to describe the human-to-human caring relationship. A prominent contemporary nursing scholar who inspired some of my later work was Gadow (1980, 1984).

These early intellectual influences were enlarged, enriched, and inspired by diverse nursing experiences and contacts with other nurses and with indigenous peoples and cultures around the world. My worldview widened to include Australia, New Zealand, Indonesia, The Republic of China, Thailand, India, and Egypt. More recently, the accumulated ideas and experiences have been expanded to include Scandinavia, England, Scotland, Canada, Portugal, Kuwait, Brazil, Japan, and Korea, among others. My work conveys a convergence and expansion of Eastern and Western beliefs, worldviews, and values. The shared aspects of humanity—life, death, suffering, caring, healing and health, and global concerns about the human-to-human connection and the condition of the planet—all are part of what I consider both universal and specific nursing phenomena, regardless of setting or country.

Thus, choosing to write about this theory with respect to a specific setting would be an arbitrary decision. Instead, mini-exemplars will be provided for each area, and a more specific focus will be directed toward the intersection of caring theory in practice and education. At this point in history, the two go hand-in-glove.

THE WORLDVIEW/COSMOLOGY FOR THE MODEL

The caring paradigm is located within a cosmology that differs from the dominant Western worldview, which treats humans as objects; separates person from self, other, nature, and the larger universe or cosmos; severs body from mind; severs spirit from both mind and body; and distinguishes health from illness, physical from metaphysical, and so on.

The context of the theory is both humanitarian and metaphysical. It calls for a return to reverence and a sense of sacredness with regard to life and human experiences, especially those related to caring and healing work with others during their most vulnerable moments of life's journey. Thus, the theory incorporates both the art and the science of nursing. Nursing is constantly expanding as a human science and is inspired by quantum physics and new models in which art and science are converging, thus incorporating and integrating diverse ways of knowing and being and doing. Because nursing phenomena are humans' and life's phenomena, multiple aspects of personal, intuitive, ethical, empirical, aesthetic, and spiritual dimensions are acknowledged as foundational to the ontological and epistemological matrix of the discipline and profession.

How Philosophical Underpinnings Relate to Practice, Education, and Research

The starting points for my work are: a value system and an explicit worldview of what it means to be human and caring when one chooses to work with others who are in need of health and healing. Caring is posited as a moral ideal and origin for nursing's professional role and "calling." In this model, caring is not just a means to a curing end, but an end in and of itself. Indeed, caring is acknowledged as representing the highest form of commitment to self, to other (Gadow, 1984), to society, to environment, and, at this point in human history, even to the universe.

This model does not consider caring as a soft, nice thing for nurses to do, or a nice way to be, in some romantic premodern sense. It posits caring knowledge and actions as a serious ontological, ethical, epistemic, and pragmatic concern for the discipline. Human consciousness is shifting toward whole-person/mind-body medicine; self-care; spiritual and existential crises; widespread interest in "alternative medicine" practitioners and options; noninvasive and nonphysical phenomena and modalities, and similar innovations. Caring and relationships based on caring are being posited as central components that the public is seeking in these healing and health outcomes.

Nursing, as a profession, exists in order to sustain caring, healing, and health where, and when, they are threatened biologically, institutionally, environmentally, or politically, by local, national, or global influences.

As a discipline, nursing has an ethical, social, and scientific responsibility to develop new theories and knowledge about caring, healing, and health practices; to teach them in education and implement them in clinical care; and to promulgate them at the ontological, epistemological, methodological, pedagogical, or praxis level.

My work thus stems from an attempt to articulate a Nursing-qua-Nursing model as a guide both to the disciplinary and professional development of nursing. As we move into the 21st century, nursing is emerging, and needs to emerge, as a mature *health* profession capable of interfacing with the *medical* profession to fulfill the highly advanced demands of *biomedical* technology.

I see modern nursing at a point in its maturity where it can step forward and claim, as its right, recognition as a distinct human caring, healing, and health profession. If it remains an extension of medicine, continuing to evolve within a Nursing-qua-Medicine model, it will not fulfill its mandate to the public, and its long effort to give society a mature caring-healing *health* profession will be vulnerable to termination.

One possibility is that another health professional group might mobilize to fulfill nursing's long-standing, but underdeveloped or unmet expectations. Another threat is that nurses will be displaced by substitute workers who will carry out the "doing tasks" that serve institutional and medical care needs, but who will not fill the huge need for professional caring-healing that nursing is poised to offer.

Without clarity of the philosophical and ethical values that are its foundation, without evolving Nursing-qua-Nursing theories, knowledge, and practice models centered on caring, healing, and *health,* nursing will potentially begin the next century within a paradigm that differs from, and often conflicts with, its own practices and heritage. Such a scenario would threaten further development of nursing's mission and accountability to the public and would interfere with the full actualization of nursing as an art and science. More importantly, this scenario would affect all levels of society and human health—personal and global, micro and macro, individual and planetary. If human caring-healing is not sustained as part of our collective values, knowledge, practices, and global mission, the survival of humankind itself is threatened. We see signs and consequences of noncaring everywhere today. Human, system, community, and ecological suffering are common worldwide, and substitution of economic concerns for person-to-person caring has become an endemic issue for nursing and a global issue for humankind.

My model of caring is located in nursing's premodern roots, yet it transcends modern industrial nursing and projects nursing into the 21st century within its own distinct paradigm.

The Caring Paradigm's Values

The components of the caring paradigm are founded on a deep respect for human existence and all living things, for the wonder and mysteries of life, and for the interconnectedness of all.

In considering what it means to be human, there is acknowledgment of the unity of mindbodyspirit/nature, and of a field of connectedness between and among persons and environments at all levels, into infinity and into the universal or cosmic level of existence.

In the words of Teilhard de Chardin (1967):

We are not human beings having a spiritual experience,
We are spiritual beings having a human experience.

The power of humans to grow and to change is an "always becoming" process; the authenticity and consciousness of *nurse* and *other* affect the process of growing, changing, and becoming.

Nonpaternalistic values relate to honoring another's becoming, autonomy, and freedom of choice; they seek to preserve personhood, human dignity, and humanity at individual and global levels.

Nurses maintain a high regard and reverence for the unfolding, subjective, inner-life world of self and other(s).

A high value is placed on subjectivity-intersubjectivity as evidenced, in a reciprocal relationship between nurse and other(s), by consciousness; intentionality; perceptions and lived experiences related to caring, healing, and health-illness conditions in a given "caring moment"; and experiences or meanings that transcend the moment and go beyond the actual experience.

Emphasis is on helping other(s), through advanced nursing caring-healing modalities, to gain more self-knowledge, self-control, and even self-healing potential, regardless of the health-illness condition.

The relationship between the nurse and other(s) is centered on with both (all) parties viewed as co-participants in the process.

Human caring is the moral ideal of nursing. The ultimate goal can be stated as: protection, enhancement, and preservation of human dignity and humanity. Caring is the moral compass or consciousness that guides our work and our reason for being.

The caring paradigm is ultimately based on the transformation of self. Beyond mere thinking, one sees possibilities for action, based on one's consciousness, intentionality, authenticity, and presence— all within a human-environment "field."

The model invokes a sense of reverence for the sacred, the spiritual, the unknown, the connectedness of all; it elicits expanded views of what it means to be human, to be healed, to be whole; it considers *person* as embodied spirit, both immanent and transcendent.

The model is transpersonal, that is, it goes beyond the personal, but it honors the validity, uniqueness, and importance of the individual as a person. Because the practitioner within a transpersonal caring-healing model seeks to be fully and authentically present, while also transcending the "ego self," the caring occasion is inter-subjective. The intentional, caring consciousness of the nurse creates a new field of possibility in a caring moment, which in turn affects the healing potential and health of both participants.

The worldview or cosmology for this caring paradigm is related to the unitary consciousness that has emerged from quantum physics and holographic views of the universe, which acknowledge that everything in the universe is connected. As we awaken to our consciousness, which is always evolving, we begin to honor and "see" the nonphysical connection, the unbroken wholeness of the universe. Although considered "new" by modern science, the concept is not new to poets and writers. Here are just two evidences of this worldview:

Within man [sic] is the soul of the whole, which is the wise silence, the universal beauty, to which every part and particle is equally related; the eternal ONE. And this deep power in which we exist and whose beatitude is all accessible to us, is not only self-sufficing and perfect in every hour, but the act of seeing and the thing seen, the seer and the spectacle, the subject and object are one.

Ralph Waldo Emerson, in The Oversoul

My brother used to ask the birds to forgive him; that sounds sense-less but it is right; for all is like the ocean, all things flow and touch each other; a disturbance in one place is felt at the other end of the world.

Fyodor Dostoyevsky, in The Brothers Karamazov

The Caring Paradigm's Assumptions (Watson, 1979/1985)

1. Care and love are the most universal, the most tremendous, and the most mysterious of cosmic forces; they comprise the primal and universal psychic energy.

2. Human needs for care and love are often overlooked; or, we know people need each other in loving and caring ways, but we do not behave well toward each other. If our humanness is to survive, we need to become more caring and loving,

thereby nourishing our humanity and evolving as civilized persons who can live together.

3. Because nursing is a caring profession, its ability to sustain its caring ideal and ideology (ethic and ethos) in education and practice will affect how humanity develops and evolves toward a moral, caring, peaceful society. In turn, nursing's contribution to society will be determined.

4. To make a beginning, we have to impose our own consciousness, moral ideal, intentionality, and will to care and love on our own behavior and awareness. We must treat ourselves with gentleness and dignity, commit to our own woundedness and healing processes. Only then will we respect and care for others with gentleness, dignity, and caring-healing consciousness.

5. Nursing has always held a human care/caring stance in regard to people, society, health-illness, and healing.

6. Caring is the essence of nursing and the most central and unifying focus for nursing practice. (Leininger, 1981).

7. Human care, at the individual, group, community, and societal levels, has received less and less emphasis in the technological systems of medical care in the late 20th century.

8. Caring values of nurses and nursing have been submerged within contemporary medical systems, which are dominated by economics. Nursing and society are, therefore, in crisis as they try to sustain human caring ideals and activities in practice. At the same time, biomedical-technological curing systems proliferate, without regard to costs or to the caring-healing and health needs of the citizenry.

9. Preservation and advancement of caring-healing and health knowledge and practices are ethical, epistemic, and clinical endeavors for all the health sciences. These issues remain particularly significant for further development of nursing science and education, and for advanced clinical care practices today and into the future.

10. Human caring can be effectively demonstrated and practiced only interpersonally; however, the process of interpersonal relationship is defined within a *transpersonal* context.

It transcends each individual and moves in concentric circles from self to other, to environment, to nature, and then to the larger universe.

11. Nursing's social, moral, and scientific contributions to humankind lie in its commitment to a human caring-healing ethic and in consciousness of its knowledge, practices, and paradigmatic matrix in theory, practice, and research endeavors.

CONTENT OF THE THEORY

Major Elements

The major conceptual elements of the original theory per se are:

- Transpersonal caring relationship
- Carative factors
- Caring occasion/Caring moment

Latent dimensions of the theory have been evolving and have emerged as more explicit components:

- Expanded views of self and person (transpersonal-mindbody-spirit oneness; embodied spirit).
- Importance of caring-healing consciousness within the human-environment field; positing of consciousness as energy.
- Phenomenal field/unitary consciousness: Unbroken wholeness and connectedness of all (subject-object-person-environment-nature-universe-all living things).
- Advanced caring-healing modalities/nursing arts.

Transpersonal Caring Relationship

Transpersonal caring was originally defined as "a human-to-human connectedness . . . each is touched by the human center of the other" (1989:131). This relationship connotes a special kind of relationship, a high regard for the whole person and his or her being-in-the-world.

When this relationship occurs within a caring consciousness, a nurse entering into the life space or phenomenal field of another person is able to detect the other person's condition of being (spirit, or soul level), feels this condition within self, and responds in such a way that the person being cared for has a release of feelings, thoughts, and tension.

Transpersonal caring can transpire in a spontaneous "caring moment" or in a caring occasion where two people have arranged to come together. Both meetings are influenced through the intersubjective nature of coming together and the phenomenal field and consciousness energy of the moment. The term *transpersonal* conveys that the connection has a spiritual dimension that is influenced by the caring consciousness of the nurse. It implies a focus on the uniqueness of self and other and the uniqueness of the phenomena wherein the coming together can be mutual and reciprocal.

Transpersonal also conveys a concern for the subjective and intersubjective meaning that is fully embodied in a uniquely personal caring moment; however, transpersonal caring also goes beyond the ego self and beyond the given moment. It moves from ego self to deeper, more spiritual, even cosmic concerns and connections that tap into healing possibilities and potentials.

Human caring and transpersonal caring both convey an ontological perspective of human "being and becoming." The ego-self has a unitary consciousness of connectedness to the embodied self (embodied spirit) of other physical persons. Transpersonal caring seeks to *embrace* the spirit or soul of those persons, through the processes of caring and healing that extend beyond ego-self and radiate to deeper connections with other, environment, nature, and the universe.

Compared to traditional modern medicine and modern nursing, this focus emerges within a different worldview. It calls forth transpersonal caring-healing practices as part of nursing's emergence within a professional and disciplinary Nursing-qua-Nursing paradigm. It is concerned with all the human experiences and conditions that affect health and illness.

Within this model, nursing can become a mature health profession and a distinct discipline within its own paradigm. Transpersonal caring calls for an authenticity of being and becoming, an ability to present as self and other in a reflective mutuality of being. The nurse then has the ability to center consciousness and intentionality on caring, healing, and wholeness, rather than on disease, illness, and complications.

Concepts such as responsivity, mutuality, intersubjectivity, expressivity, and engagement of nurse with other, even in a spontaneous moment, become critical for a mature caring-healing professional. The human caring "ontological competencies" of the nurse (and of other health professionals) become as essential as the "technological competencies" that are currently defining or directing the advancement of modern nursing and medicine.

Within the model of transpersonal caring, the nurse will attempt to stay within the other's frame of reference, to join in a mutual search for meaning and wholeness of being, to potentiate comfort measures, pain control, a sense of well-being, or spiritual transcendence of suffering. Consciousness of new ways of being can give meaning to the experience of suffering while living. The person is considered valid and whole, regardless of illness, or disease. That intact wholeness, the constant reintegration of mindbodyspirit, being fully immanent, is paradoxically transcendent.

A transpersonal caring relationship depends on (Watson, 1985/1988c, p. 63):

- The moral commitment, intentionality, and consciousness needed to protect, enhance, promote, and potentiate human dignity, wholeness, and healing, wherein a person creates or cocreates his or her own meaning for existence, healing, wholeness, and caring.
- Orientation of the nurse's intent, will, and consciousness toward affirming the subjective/intersubjective significance of the person; a search to sustain mindbodyspirit unity and I–Thou versus I–It relationships.
- The nurse's ability to realize, accurately detect, and connect with the inner condition (spirit) of another; actions, words, behaviors, cognition, body language, feelings, intuition, thought, senses, the energy field gestalt, and so on, all contribute to the interconnection.

- The nurse's ability to assess and realize another's condition of being-in-the-world and to feel a union with the other. This ability is translated—via movements, gestures, facial expressions, procedures, information, touch, sound, verbal expressions, and other scientific, aesthetic, and human means of communication—into nursing-art acts wherein the nurse responds to, attends to, or reflects the condition of the other. Drawn from the ontological caring-consciousness stance and basic competencies of the nurse, this ability expands and translates into advanced caring-healing modalities, nursing arts, advanced nursing therapeutics, healing arts, and so on.
- The caring-healing modalities potentiate harmony, wholeness, and comfort, and promote inner healing by releasing some of the disharmony and blocked energy that interfere with the natural healing processes.
- The nurse's own life history and previous experiences. Opportunities, studies, consciousness of having lived through or experienced human feelings and various human conditions, or of having imagined others' feelings in various circumstances, are valuable contributors. To some degree, the necessary knowledge and sensitivity can be gained through work with other cultures, study of the humanities (art, drama, and literature), and exploration of one's own values, beliefs, and relationship with self. Other facilitators are: personal growth experiences such as psychotherapy, meditation, bioenergetics work, and spiritual awakening. Continuous growth is related to personal growth, maturity, development of the nurse's (transpersonal) self, sensitivity to others, and deep inner experiences that connect with a universal field of consciousness.

Carative Factors

Transpersonal caring is actualized and "grounded" through ten carative factors that characterize a human-to-human nursing caring transaction within a given caring occasion. The ten carative factors serve as a guide to the "core" (in contrast to the "trim") of nursing. Core refers to those aspects of nursing that actually potentiate therapeutic healing processes for both the one caring and the one being cared for. The core of nursing is grounded in the philosophy, science, and art of caring (which is posited to be intrinsically related to healing). The trim refers to the practice setting, procedures, functional tasks, specialized clinical focus, technology, techniques, and specific medical/disease-oriented services surrounding the diverse orientations and preoccupations of nursing. The trim, however, is in no way entirely expendable. Nurses throughout time have practiced these carative factors in conjunction with the trim activities, without naming them as such.

Nevertheless, in this caring model, the carative factors are posited as the primary ingredients for effective nursing practice. Each nurse, depending on his or her educational background, clinical focus, and personal orientation, masters an approach to nursing care that incorporates carative factors. An advanced awareness of consciously operating within a nursing caring model helps to promote nursing's practice and sustain nursing within its own paradigm. In other words, the carative factors are not "new" to nursing; most nurses already use them in their practice. But they are less often named or "seen," and they are practiced on the margin of the dominant institutional medical care model.

The caring model and carative factors provide a language, structure, and order for nursing education and practice. Vocabulary and choice of language become increasingly important at this point in our history, wherein language defines us.

Postmodern writers remind us that, without one's own language, "You do not exist." Throughout history, nursing has adopted or adapted others' languages for nursing phenomena. Thus, nursing, as the largest health care profession, ironically is not often seen as distinct in its own right. Instead, nursing is seen as an extension of modern medicine.

Even nursing's most contemporary language for advanced practice roles and nursing diagnosis is a subset of Western medicine. It is not nursing's language that names and describes human experience phenomena and caring-healing processes of human health.

In addition to providing language for nursing phenomena, the carative factors help define nursing knowledge and practices as distinct from, but complementary with, the curing knowledge and practices associated with traditional medicine.

As one interacts with and matures within this model, it becomes increasingly evident that the caring-healing dimensions of nursing both parallel and intersect with what is now commonly referred to as mind-body medicine: noninvasive, nonintrusive, natural healing modalities; the alternative complementary medicine frameworks that are common among the public today.

My model is congruent with recent reports on health care reform, which call for "centrality of caring-healing relationships" as the foundation for all health professional education and practice reform.

The central task of health professions education—in nursing, medicine, dentistry, public health, pharmacy, psychology, social work, and the allied health professions—must be to help students, faculty, and practitioners learn how to form caring, healing relationships with patients, and their communities, and with each other, and with themselves . . . the knowledge, skills, and values necessary for effective relationships. . . . Developing practitioners mature as reflective learners and professionals who understand the patient as a person, recognize and deal with multiple contributions to health and illness, and understand the essential nature of healing relationships. (Pew-Fetzer Task Force Report, 1994 p. 39)

The ten carative factors, which provide a structure for such recommendations, consist of the following:

1. Forming a humanistic-altruistic system of values.
2. Enabling and sustaining faith-hope.
3. Being sensitive to self and others.
4. Developing a helping-trusting, caring relationship (seeking transpersonal connection).
5. Promoting and accepting the expression of positive and negative feelings and emotions.
6. Engaging in creative, individualized, problem-solving caring processes.
7. Promoting transpersonal teaching-learning.
8. Attending to supportive, protective, and/or corrective mental, physical, societal, and spiritual environments.
9. Assisting with gratification of basic human needs while preserving human dignity and wholeness.

10. Allowing for, and being open to, existential-phenomenological and spiritual dimensions of caring and healing that cannot be fully explained scientifically through modern Western medicine.

It is important to point out that, although the ten carative factors provide the skeletal foundation for the original work, they are embedded within a worldview that is transpersonal, dynamic, and evolving. The carative factors are not intended as a checklist or a prescription, but as a philosophical and conceptual guide toward a model of caring for nursing. They are intended to help define elements of nursing within its own paradigm, regardless of specific medical diagnoses and treatment demands.

The carative factors also serve as a foundation for building and developing advanced practices and caring modalities for healing and health processes and outcomes. The model accommodates traditional medical protocols and traditional functional tasks of modern nursing, while remaining oriented to nursing's mature development.

(For the content and description of the carative factors, see Watson, 1979/1985, 1985/1988c, 1989; also see Fawcett, 1993, for a brief overview of the carative factors.)

Caring Occasion/Caring Moment

A caring occasion occurs whenever nurse and other(s) come together with their unique life histories and phenomenal field in a human-to-human transaction. The coming together in a given moment becomes a focal point in space and time. Experience and perception take place, but the actual caring occasion has a greater field of its own. The process goes beyond itself, yet arises from aspects of itself that become part of the life history of each person, as well as part of some larger, deeper, more complex pattern of life (Watson, 1985/1988c, p. 59).

The actual caring occasion, or caring moment, involves action and choice by both the nurse and the other. The moment of coming together presents them with the opportunity to decide how to *be* in the relationship—what to do with the moment. If the caring moment is transpersonal, each feels a connection with the other, and the spirits of both create openness. The occasion then has the ability to expand the field of possibilities and the sense of being connected with another human's experience.

> . . . we learn from one another how to be human by identifying ourselves with others, finding their dilemmas in ourselves. What we all learn from it is self-knowledge. The self we learn about . . . is every self; it is universal—the human self. We learn to recognize ourselves in others . . . [it] keeps alive our common humanity and avoids reducing self or other to the moral and actual status of object. (Watson, 1985/1988, pp. 59–60)

Caring (Healing) Consciousness

A holographic dynamic of transpersonal caring (healing), within a caring moment, is manifest within a field of consciousness.

The transpersonal dimensions of a caring occasion are affected by the nurse's consciousness in the caring moment, which in turn affects the field dynamic of the transaction. The gestalt of transpersonal caring and the role of consciousness with respect to caring and healing have been discussed within a holographic framework as follows:

- *The whole caring-healing consciousness is contained within a single caring moment.*
- *The one caring and the one being cared for are interconnected; the caring-healing process is connected with other humans and [draws on] the higher energy of the universe.*
- *The caring-healing consciousness of the nurse is communicated to the one being cared for.*
- *Caring-healing consciousness exists through and transcends time and space and can be dominant over physical illness. (Watson, 1992: 148)*

Within the holographic context for transpersonal caring and healing, it is acknowledged that the process is relational and connected; transcends self, time, space, and physical dominance; and is intersubjective with transcendent possibilities that go beyond the given caring occasion.

Connections: Caring-Healing Consciousness and Energy

Emerging aspects of the roles of consciousness, energy, health, and well-being have resulted from quantum physics and newer models of science. The following excerpts from Zukav (1990), a physicist, help us to reconsider the significance of one's (caring-healing) consciousness with respect to caring professionals and aspects of mind-bodyspirit health, wholeness, and harmony.

> *A thought is energy, or Light, that has been shaped by consciousness. (p. 105)*

> *Emotions are currents of energy with different frequencies. When you choose to replace a lower frequency current, such as anger, with a higher frequency current, such as forgiveness (caring) . . . affection, love, compassion . . . you raise the frequency of your Light. (p. 94)*

> *If your thoughts are thoughts that draw low-frequency energy currents to you, your physical and emotional attitudes will deteriorate, and emotional or physical disease will follow, whereas thoughts that draw high-frequency energy currents to you create physical and emotional health. (p. 95)*

> *Lower frequency systems pull energy from higher frequency systems. We say, for example, a depressed patient is "draining," or that he or she "sucks up energy." A system of sufficiently high frequency (caring-healing consciousness) will soothe, or calm, or refresh because of the quality of Light. (p. 95)*

> *If you (we) are unaware of y/our emotions and thoughts (y/our consciousness and intentionality, for example) y/our frequency will be lowered by—you (we) will lose energy to—a system of lower frequency than y/our own. (p. 95)*

> *By choosing y/our (consciousness) . . . and by selecting y/our emotional currents, you will release, and will reinforce, . . . the quality of your Light (pp. 94-95).*

The caring-healing consciousness of a caring moment opens up a higher, deeper energy field of consciousness that has metaphysical and spiritual potentialities for healing and goes beyond the separate ego self and separate body (physical) self. Transpersonal caring has the capacity to expand human consciousness, transcend the moment, and potentiate healing and a sense of well-being—a sense of being reintegrated, more connected, more whole.

Based on these notions of caring consciousness and energy, nursing, *collectively,* with its caring consciousness, has the potential to enable individuals, systems, and humankind to move toward higher-frequency possibilities that offer greater harmony, wholeness, health, and spiritual evolution, while sustaining increasing diversity. Individually, one's caring consciousness can help to shift the field of recovery for self and others.

PRACTICAL IMPLEMENTATIONS OF THE CARING MODEL

As noted in the introduction, at one level, my model is considered philosophically and ethically foundational to all areas of nursing practice, education, and research. No one focus for its "application" becomes a favored exemplar, because it has been used as a guide for all of these areas. At another level, as it evolves in maturity of ideas and actions, it calls forth advanced clinical and educational practices for its "application" while, at the same time, requiring additional study, development, and research.

As an aside, it is important to acknowledge that this work can be read, taught, learned about, studied, researched, and even practiced; however, to truly "get it," one has to personally *experience* it—interact and grow within the philosophy and intention of the model. Nevertheless, it can be and is being "applied" across a spectrum, in varying degrees.

I am open to others' experimenting with the model, altering it, and engaging in it at whatever level they can locate themselves within its ideas—whether as a philosophy, an ethic, an ontology, a paradigm, an abstract or middle-range theory, a model, or a specific theory. Moreover, it can be considered a bridge between traditional and emerging paradigms (e.g., interactive to unitary transformative) within nursing and health sciences generally.

If one chooses to interact with this caring paradigm and specific aspects of the caring model for any one setting, the following critical questions must be considered:

- Is there congruence between (a) the values and assumptions in the model that form the foundation for the philosophy, ethic, and ethos of the "theory" and (b) the given individual nurse, group, system, organization, curriculum, patient population, clinical administrative setting, or other entity, that is considering its use?

- What is the perspective on human life and on how humans (both nurses and others) grow and change? What answer would be given to this question, derived from the statement by Teilhard de Chardin: Are these humans having a spiritual experience, or are they spiritual beings having a human experience?

    (One does not have to fully answer this rhetorical question, but it can guide one's worldview, belief system, and view of humans; ultimately, one's view of humans will direct all other aspects of professional nursing, consciously or unconsciously.)

- Are those engaged with the model interested in their own personal evolution as spiritual beings? Are they seeking authentic connections and caring-healing relationships with others?

- Are those involved "conscious" of their caring or noncaring consciousness and its positive or negative potential at the individual or system level? Are they interested in and committed to expanding their caring consciousness to self and other, to the environment, ecology, nature, and the wider universe? Are they moving in consciousness from lower-frequency thought systems to higher-frequency thought systems?

- Are those involved interested in shifting their focus from a Nursing-qua-Medicine model to a Nursing-qua-Nursing model, located within a caring-healing paradigm?

Other questions practitioners and educators can ask, when choosing the most compatible model to suit their practice are:

- What sense can we make of the ideas and concepts within the model for our personal practice and the population we serve?

- Do the values and assumptions in the model match our values, beliefs, and assumptions about the nature of our educational and practice goals?
- Does the model work for us (a continuous critical question)?
- How does this work help us in what we are trying to achieve with our self, our patients, the community, and the broader health care system?
- How can we interpret this model for our curriculum? Our practice?
- What sort of personal and professional development do we need before we can practically, philosophically, and intellectually implement this model?

MINI-EXEMPLARS OF THE MODEL IN ACTION

Nursing Education

The human caring theory is, and has had, both a direct and an indirect influence on nursing and health science curricula and pedagogy, and on health sciences education generally. In numerous academic programs, in the United States and in other countries, the model is being used as a major curricular structure, a theoretical model, and/or an educational, philosophical, and operational paradigm for department-/school-wide educational programs. "Caring" is now commonly incorporated at some level within most nursing curricula in the United States. If my work is not used as a guide to the actual curriculum and coursework, it is among those usually included for study.

The Ideal Educational Model for the Caring Paradigm. The human caring theory can be used at different levels, but, taken to its full educational actualization, it places nursing in a mature academic-professional-educational model. Ideally, these facets of the model would be fulfilled as:

- Academic: Postbaccalaureate graduate level.
- Professional: Advanced practice in nursing and as an expert professional in caring-healing and health.

- Education: "Attending nurse" status, working alongside other members of the health team, while assuming responsibility for the caring-healing focus of care.

This advanced, rigorous, educational-practice model would merit a graduate degree in nursing, preferably the nursing doctorate (N.D.).

Such an educational-practice program prepares the nurse to advance clinically within a Nursing-qua-Nursing model. It takes the nurse beyond the traditional nurse practitioner responsibilities, and it incorporates advanced caring-healing modalities and nursing arts therapeutics into the educational and practice foundations. Nurses trained in the current model for hospital nursing, and the traditional medical services orientation for primary care, will need additional professional development and continuing education to practice within this collaborative educational-practice model. The advanced nurse may not always deliver the care directly; in some instances, he or she will oversee, coordinate, and mediate the continuous caring-healing health care needs of individuals, families, and groups. The nurses will practice wherever the patients/clients are located: in and outside of institutions, schools, homes, clinics, and community settings. The vision for this model projects the future: posthospital nursing delivered to people individually and collectively within a continuous care model. In this educational-practice model, patients could bring their own nurse to a hospital to assume responsibility for "attending" to a full range of their individualized caring-healing needs, including mediating among multiple providers and systems, and ensuring continuity of their care needs.

Caring theory in education is intrinsically tied to new models of nursing practice. For both education and practice, caring theory calls for transformative models that are consistent with a 21st-century perspective on the changing nature of science, mind-body medicine, and nonphysical caring-healing modalities that potentiate self-care, self-knowledge, and self-healing. Nurses will need to assume new roles as caring-focused communicators of clinical care-community-education; as practitioners, they will need hands-on advanced caring-healing knowledge and skills, and the capacity to operate in a holographic work "space," via international communication networks, informatics systems, and closed-circuit client/other practitioners/team networks.

At the N.D. level, the University of Colorado is implementing a national model curriculum in caring-healing and health; it is guided by the caring paradigm and my work, but its approach is multitheoretical and broad-based. This model curriculum was funded by the Helene Fuld Health Trust as an experimental postbaccalaureate nursing doctorate program. The program, its students, and its first graduates (in 1994) are being comprehensively evaluated.

This curricular work and model program, as well as general aspects of caring curricula and nursing education have been described in several publications (Bevis & Watson, 1989; Leininger & Watson, 1990; Sakalys & Watson, 1985, 1986; Watson, 1985/1988c, 1987, 1988b, 1988d, 1990; Watson & Bevis, 1990; Watson & Phillips, 1992).

Common Educational Uses of the Caring Paradigm. The caring paradigm, as a model, is not limited to implementing the full graduate-level N.D. model; it remains relevant to nursing at all other educational levels. For example, it has applicability, at varying degrees of depth and scope, in technical and entry-level programs: L.P.N., Diploma, A.D., and B.S. Its present uses and future possibilities include:

- An introductory framework for orienting students to a foundational model for professional nursing practice.
- An overall framework for considering patient-/person-centered care and caring consciousness as a central philosophy, ethic, or ethos for all nursing practice (regardless of level of preparation).
- A model for advancing clinical practice by fostering educational progression from technical focus to mature professional expertise.
- A curricular framework whereby the philosophy and ethic of caring guide content that is organized around the ten carative factors. For example, in some programs, the carative factors are used as threads or commonalities throughout each course; in others, the carative factors are a matrix for course content: courses focus, in different depth, on particular carative factors while attempting to sustain the "whole caring model" in each course or each part of the curriculum.

- A philosophical and content (organized around the carative factors) guide to teaching nursing's caring-healing arts, and to organizing caring-healing arts "labs" as part of teaching nursing "skills," "foundations," and "essentials."
- A philosophical, conceptual, and theoretical guide to professional practice at the B.S. level and above.
- A specific theory of caring to study as part of the extant philosophy, theories, and knowledge of nursing that help to comprise the disciplinary matrix for professional education, practice, and research; a core concept for analysis in both undergraduate and graduate programs.

As a guide for nursing education, whether at the entry or advanced level, this theory orients students to a Nursing-qua-Nursing paradigm that is consistent with its heritage, with the finest of its most ancient and contemporary caring-healing practices, and with the art and artistry of nursing practice. The human focus is central to both pedagogy and practice.

Educationally, this model calls for more integration of the arts and humanities into nursing education (and practice); it allows for progression into a more congruent human focus for redefining nursing arts. Human skills are paramount and are equal to technological skills with respect to caring and healing.

Greater use of art, music, sound, literature, story, poetry, drama, and movement, and greater acknowledgment of the bioenergetics models that help to reintegrate mindbodyspirit through nursing arts and therapeutics, are encouraged in the model. The benefits can be reframed as: conscious and intentional use of auditory, visual, olfactory, sensory, gustatory, tactile, cognitive, and interpersonal communication; and consciousness modalities as foundational and preparatory for advanced professional nursing practice within a caring-healing paradigm.

The model incorporates traditional nursing skills and techniques, along with advanced practitioner skills, within the context of human caring values, ethics, knowledge, and relationships.

The advanced caring-healing modalities or advanced nursing therapeutics that result incorporate natural healing modalities (along with traditional medical treatment needs) for offering comfort measures, pain control, symptom management, self-care modalities (which potentiate a sense of well-being), self-control, and so on.

Traditional nursing skills can be redefined within a nursing-arts, caring-healing model as *advanced practice nursing*. Elements include, for example: therapeutic massage, intentional touch, therapeutic touch, healing touch, aromatherapy (and/or use of essential oils and other substances) to promote olfactory pleasures, soothing, and calming sensations; and intentional introduction of sound, music, art, jounaling, movement, relaxation, and visualization, among other untapped nursing-art acts that reside within a Nursing-qua-Nursing caring-healing model for both education and practice. The model requires a transformation and a dramatic shift for advanced nursing practice. It also has profound implications for nursing research, cost-effective care, clinical care, and quality-of-life outcome studies.

Practice/Administrative Implementation

Full actualization of this model requires new ways of thinking and being. At one level, the model is obvious and perhaps already in action; others may consider it too remote, abstract, and ethereal, however. At whatever level it is approached, the model is always fragile and threatened because it requires a personal, social, moral, and spiritual engagement of self. Thus, users of the model face a radical transformation of traditional professional relationships and ways of thinking about nursing as "doing." As a basis for practice, the model invites openness and encourages new possibilities to be forthcoming from the practitioners and recipients alike. The transpersonal aspect involves the participants in cocreating the model's emergence. It is not easy to adopt such a professional model for practice, especially if one engages in nursing as a technical employee of an institution and has not made a commitment to humanity as one's life's work and service.

A model of human caring, with its need for ethics, emotions, compassion, knowledge, wisdom, intentions, and so on, requires continual engagement and continual personal development and growth.

However, just as the model can be engaged in at the concrete level, using the carative factors as a clinical care guide, it can also be engaged in at a more transpersonal level, using advanced caring-healing practices. Moreover, for some institutions, the model serves as a formal philosophy for an entire health care system: a hospital, a unit, or a given clinical population (e.g., the elderly, persons with AIDS, or the chronically ill); a given setting (e.g., hospice or home); in-patient critical care; pediatric care; transplant care; and so on. The theory has been used as a guide to practice, rather than as a specific "theory-based" practice model.

In general, examples of how the theory has directly influenced nursing practice are increasing in the literature. It has been reported to be the foundation for clinical nursing care in the following hospitals in Canada:

Baycrest Centre for Geriatric Care, Toronto, Ontario
Doctors' Hospital, Toronto, Ontario (General Medical)
Princess Margaret Hospital, Toronto, Ontario (Children's Hospital)
The Montreal General Hospital, Montreal, Quebec
The Rehabilitation Hospital of Montreal, Montreal, Quebec
Université de Montreal, Faculté des Sciences Infirmières

Denver Nursing Project in Human Caring. In the United States, the most prominent example is the Denver Nursing Project in Human Caring, a clinical demonstration project of the University of Colorado School of Nursing and the Center for Human Caring. The project has become an international model for theory-guided practice based on both the philosophical foundation of the caring model and the actual theory concepts such as transpersonal caring and the use of the carative factors. Although this model was originally strictly "Watson's theory" in practice (and it still is, in the broadest sense), as I have worked with and observed the implementation, I have encouraged nurses and other health team members to consider it a caring-based practice (guided by the philosophy, ethic, and theoretical constructs of the carative factors) but not be bound by it; rather, they should use it as a mutually informing process, wherein they interact with the theory rather than "applying it" in some preconceived conforming way. This way of working with the theory allows theory-guided

practice and practice-guided theory to intersect. Moreover, by
working with the theory in this broader sense, different practitioners can engage in multitheoretical perspectives while still
sharing and staying within a common paradigm that embraces the
caring-healing process and relations.

The Denver Nursing Project in Human Caring was established in
1988 as an outpatient center for clients with HIV infection/AIDS.
Since that time, the Center has hosted more than 21,000 client visits. Currently, it has more than 300 active clients. The sponsorship
of the nurse-directed Center and theory-based practice model is
shared by three Denver hospitals (Denver Veterans Hospital, University Hospital, and Denver General Hospital) and serves as a clinical
demonstration of the University of Colorado School of Nursing and
the Center for Human Caring. HIV-infected persons are eligible,
whether they are medically referred or self-referred.

The Center provides blood transfusions, IV fluids, pentamidine
treatment, and other direct medically supportive care services; however, the main focus is on caring-based practices for all the nursing
and health care offered. For example, there are numerous educational and supportive services (individual and group); alternative-
complementary caring-healing modalities, such as massage,
therapeutic touch, art therapy, poetry, and journal writing; aerobics
classes; exercise physiology programs; dental screening; lunches
and other opportunities for clients to be with friends and with caring professionals in a positive healing environment.

Caring relationships are central: staff-staff, staff-client, client-
client, and staff-client-community. Meaningful client involvement is
manifest through caring partnerships between and among staff (and
volunteers) and clients. A Client Advisory Committee is part of the
system of care. Clients prepare and disseminate a newsletter, are actively engaged in fund raising in the community, and share in the
center's educational programs.

The Denver Nursing Project has been federally funded since
1990 by the Department of Health and Human Services (DHHS) Division of Nursing. The Center has been recognized for the quality
of its services and programs by the AIDS Lobby for Better Living,
Region VIII of the DHHS, Sigma Theta Tau International, the Annual Rocky Mountain Regional Conference on HIV Disease, and

the 31st Annual Excellence in Government Awards Program. At the same time, the Center has also been the subject of numerous publications, and some videos documenting the experimental clinical demonstration project.

Baycrest Centre for Geriatric Care, Toronto, Ontario.   Eileen Cappell, Director of Innovative Nursing Services at Baycrest, obtained funding from the Canadian Health Ministry for developing, implementing, and evaluating a caring-theory-based practice model for nursing and allied health personnel at Baycrest. Watson's theory of human caring is used as the guide for approximately 650 RNs, RNAs, and health care aides. Baycrest states in the institutional literature that "Watson's theory of nursing, Nursing: Human Science and Human Care, provides the theoretical foundation for all aspects of nursing at the Centre."

The implementation process, which proceeded unit by unit, included formal and informal educational and clinical in-service programs and initiatives. For example, early on, a process referred to as "conceptual mapping" (Cappell, 1994, p. 12) was begun, to establish the fit among the problem, the innovation, and the organization. Cappell describes this process as labor-intensive, in that, during this period, the staff reviewed eight nursing theories before selecting Watson's theory to guide their practices at Baycrest. All areas of nursing and all levels of practice were represented in the review of the various theories.

The criteria that Baycrest established in selecting the conceptual-philosophical fit included the values and beliefs within the theory that supported an abiding view of care/caring already held by the institution and the staff. Other values within the theory were reviewed for possible adoption and promotion. For example, Cappell (1994) identified Watson's views of "high respect for life, and the power of humans to grow and change" as being important in caring for elders because:

> this value would empower us to see the potential for people to grow and change despite age and/or infirmity. Explicit adoption of this value would allow us as gerontological nurses to be hopeful, and to approach people with a sense of optimism and purpose. (p. 13)

Other considerations in adopting and implementing a theory-guided practice included: worldview with respect to concept of health and Watson's view of the unity and harmony of mindbody-spirit.

> *Defining health in this way helps nurses see their care as active and purposeful toward achieving the goal of promoting health (harmony, unity). Some of the process included asking themselves questions about their worldview and key concepts which affect their practice. (p. 13)*

Cappell describes the implementation phase as the first step toward refining or modifying the theory to fit the organization. For example, at Baycrest, the theory was geared toward older people who live in the long-term care institution.

> *Theory is meant to be lived and experienced. Modify the theory in the ways that will let you live a caring philosophy. In turn, by living caring theory, you will engage in a form of action research which will lead to enhancing our understanding and knowledge of caring theory. (p. 14)*

During this stage, project coordinators were involved with organizational unit-specific responsibilities and with overseeing the implementation. This process ensures staff involvement and commitment, within an open system, to the choice of model.

In teaching the caring theory, the Baycrest team sought to let the theory guide them; for example, innovative teaching methods, such as poetry and music, were used. Interactive methods were designed to encourage self-reflection and increased self-awareness. Caring for staff became an important aspect of this process.

Regular meetings to sustain the process were also found essential. At Baycrest, regular sessions were held for at least six months to help staff reflect on how the theory was manifest in their practice. During this phase, the carative factors were used to guide the establishment of a caring relationship. Other caring modalities—for example, therapeutic touch, gardening, and aesthetically enriched environments—were also pursued as part of advancing clinical care practices.

Cappell pointed out that, from her experience and work, and consistent with the theory:

Implementation of caring theory should not be limited to caring occasions between nurses and clients. Rather, it should be used to help staff feel cared for as well, because this is foundational for being able to care for others. (p. 15)

Cappell noted other happenings from the Baycrest experience. Once the theory is implemented and introduced as a conscious mode of practicing, it moves beyond the individual and unit level to middle management, senior management, and other disciplines in the system.

Consistent with the theory, the management/administrative philosophy at Baycrest is especially facilitative. Decentralized decision making and supportive leadership also include regular involvement of families and clients in unit-based quality care groups.

As a teaching facility, Baycrest Centre is affiliated with the University of Toronto for both research and education, and with other teaching institutions such as McMaster University, Seneca College, and Humber College. Undergraduate and graduate-level educational/research opportunities are offered.

The nursing facility at Baycrest evaluates the activities of all its programs; in this case, research was done on the effect of theory-based practice on the quality of nurses' work life and patient care indicators. More recently, there have been some initiatives to integrate the caring theory model into total quality management (TQM) programs and outcome indicators. To date, while a formal evaluation progresses, the project is considered a success in advancing the clinical practice of nurses and allied health personnel.

Multiple approaches for implementing caring-theory-guided practice were acknowledged by Baycrest to be consistent with TQM as well. Recognizing staff as experts, celebrating success, viewing problems as opportunities, giving staff feedback on the whole project, and valuing staff's role in the project and the organization were cited for compatibility with TQM.

As a result of the enormous commitment and continuous support and processing the caring model gained there, Baycrest has become a model of caring theory in action throughout the world. In 1994–1995, Baycrest became a formal International Clinical Affiliate of the University of Colorado Center for Human Caring, a member of the network of the Colorado Center and its national/international affiliates and collaborative partners in others parts of the world. As an active partner in networking for future international developments in clinical caring research and consultation, Baycrest hosts visitors and participates in shaping new global directions with other international affiliates. It is an international clinical exemplar for caring theory in practice throughout an entire system.

Visitors to Baycrest will find the model evident, not only with respect to direct patient care, but in colleague-to-colleague and staff-to-management relationships and processes for problem solving. The concept of caring in action at several levels is manifest throughout the culture of the system and in collaborative relationships with other disciplines, which have, in turn, become interested in working within a shared caring paradigm for the good of the whole.

Cappell and the Nursing Innovative Team and Staff had the foresight to use the theory as a guide in their implementation work. For example, whenever they would get "stuck" or feel that their efforts were not progressing, or when distractions such as budget cuts, staff cuts, and changes occurred (and they did, during the implementation work), they reported that they would "always go back to the theory, to see if they could be guided on how to proceed." According to their communication with me, the theory, in those trying instances, got them back on center course with each other and with the values they were attempting to consciously live out.

From Cappell's (1994) extensive pioneering work at Baycrest, she concluded that, although the commitment is enormous, "caring theory promises to be a central and unifying force for nursing which in turn will lead to tremendous personal, professional, and societal gains" (p. 17).

Rockford Health System, University of Illinois at Chicago, College of Nursing Rockford Program.   A more recent caring-theory-based practice model has been funded at the Rockford Health System in Illinois. Dr. Paula Christensen, the project director, initiated the project activities in the spring of 1995. She is implementing the theory through a series of workshop/in-service programs structured around nurses' specific interests and related to different aspects of how the theory can manifest itself in the professional development of the nursing staff. For example, the staff first participates in a general orientation to the theory, its concepts, and the carative factors. Personalized, interactive, innovative, and aesthetic learning, as well as cognitive and experiential processes, are then explored. Thereafter, each nurse has the opportunity to select advanced caring-theory-based learning/clinical practice experiences among the following options:

Caring competencies

Therapeutic presence	Authenticity/Self-reflection
Intuition	Centeredness/Mindfulness
Active listening	Connectedness/Openness

Caring modalities

Therapeutic Touch	Journaling
Music	Meditation
Guided imagery	Relaxation
Therapeutic massage	Humor
Drawing	

Caring strategies

Caring for the caregiver	Ethics of caring
Communities of caring	Aesthetics and caring
Caring and leadership	Meaning (making it part of work)

The Rockford project is active at this time and is another example of Watson's caring theory being used to influence nursing practice both through professional development/education and in direct clinical care programs. In its creative approaches to implementing the work, the Rockford project parallels the two exemplars described earlier, and which include caring-healing modalities for advancing patient care in traditional in-patient settings and in a nursing clinic setting.

Other Implementations

In practice

Children's Hospital, Denver, Colorado
Del Webb Hospital, Sun City West, Arizona
Englewood Hospital, Englewood, New Jersey
Holmes Regional Medical Center, Florida
King's Daughter Hospital, Ashland, Kentucky
Medical Clinics of Houston, Houston, Texas
Mt. Carmel Hospital, Columbus, Ohio
Winter Haven Hospital, Winter Haven, Florida

It is impossible to be informed and updated on all the clinical initiatives where nurses are using the theory as a guide to their individual practices, but some examples have emerged in the literature regarding specific populations and diverse settings.

Individuals. Aucoin-Gallant (1990), in describing the use of carative factors in nursing practice, indicated benefits for both caregivers and care receivers: "clients and families developing a sense of responsibility and control over illness-induced stress. For the nurse . . . a source of motivation and job satisfaction."

Sithichoke-Rattan (1989) also reported using the theory for preterm infants and their parents.

In Clinically Based Practice and Research. Lemmer's (1991) study of parental perceptions of caring following a perinatal death found five of the carative factors supported with this population.

For her part, Schindel-Martin (1990, 1991) conducted qualitative studies on clinical caring, guided by the carative factors, with persons undergoing long-term hemodialysis and adults with polycystic kidney disease. Her work supports Watson's theory, especially with respect to the interpersonal (caring) relationship.

Clayton (1989) reported using Watson's caring theory in both practice and research with an elderly population. She found that the carative factors guided practice with elders: the nurses' feelings regarding their own emotions and sensitivity to elders were heightened both prior to and following the caring interaction. Other findings revealed the existence of a helping-trusting relationship; elders themselves reported that the behaviors of nurses (practicing within the caring model) "opened the possibility for trust" (p. 250).

Briefly, the carative factors created a supportive, protective, and "permissive" environment that preserved the uniqueness of each individual. Existential forces were expressed through a recognition (by the elders) that the nurses understood and appreciated their situations and their unique struggle with institutionalization.

Although Clayton (1989) reported that these clinical findings were congruent with the theory of caring, she also noted the need for additional research. New methodologies and multiple approaches are necessary for expanding our understanding of the caring phenomena.

Focussing on the experience of spirituality with well adults, Burns (1991) found congruence between "the construct of transpersonal caring, proposed by Watson to involve two phenomenal fields (humans with unique life experiences) coming together during an actual caring occasion and experiencing the presence of the spirit of both" and the participants in the study (p. 149). She discussed the merging of phenomenal fields as being "supported by all 22 experiences with the possible configurations: human with human; human with God (or whatever level one uses for transcendent being); or human with human with transcendent" (p. 150). In general, Burns concluded that the concepts (e.g., human center with energy and power of its own; transpersonal intersubjectivity—two phenomenal fields coming together; transcendence; caring expanding the limits of openness and human capacities; and presence of the "theory of transpersonal caring") were supported in her "phenomenological study of spirituality" (p. 151). She recommended that the focus of the theory of transpersonal caring needs be expanded to include the study of the components of spirituality, particularly the depth experience, as it occurs in the everyday living of persons. Finally, she acknowledged that the transpersonal caring process "must be investigated as it relates to wellness and health promotion activities of persons" (p. 152).

Duffy (1990, 1992) explored the impact of nurse caring on patient outcomes. Based on her critical care experiences and interests, she measured the relationships between nurse caring behaviors and selected outcomes of patient satisfaction, health status, length of stay, and nursing care costs in hospitalization medical and/or surgi-cal patients. Using a descriptive correlational research design, she studied 86 subjects. Data were collected via (a) the Caring Assess-ment Tool (designed by the researcher); (b) the Patient Satisfaction Visual Analog Scale; (c) Sickness Impact Profile; (d) Medicus Patient Classification Tool; and (e) Patient Information Form for demo-graphic and descriptive data.

She reported using Watson's theory of human care as the theoret-ical framework for the study. Her work specifically identified the caring behaviors of nurses as they related to patient satisfaction, which she acknowledged as a new finding. (1992, p. 128). She did not find significant relationships between nurse caring behaviors and health status, length of stay, or medical care costs which, while related in the right direction, were not statistically significant. She discussed the notion that nurse caring behaviors might be a possible predictor of patient satisfaction; none of the other variables in her study were correlated with patient satisfaction.

Duffy concluded that full use of the carative factors in daily nurse–patient interactions provides a foundation for nursing prac-tice. Noting that use of these factors requires a commitment on the part of the hospital nurse, she advised faculty to review their con-ceptual base and modify it to fit a more interpersonal human inter-acting approach.

Faculty should role-model the carative factors often through cre-ative, sensitizing activities with students. Requiring students to master the carative factors, [as well as] procedural techniques, will reinforce the importance of these practices for students in every-day worklife. (1992, p. 130)

Nursing administrators also need to find ways to facilitate caring practices in their staff; nurses who supervise other nurses must use the carative factors in their daily practice as well. Duffy noted that the carative factors also serve administrators as a conceptual and operational model for practice, helping to develop a culture of car-ing within the institution.

McNamara (1995) reported on the use of carative factors in all phases of perioperative nursing. (This was the first formal study in the literature, to my knowledge, of using Watson's theory to research caring practices of perioperative nurses.) She used a qualitative, descriptive methodology and found caring behaviors being identified with conscious and unconscious patients in the preoperative, intraoperative, and postoperative periods. The nurse subjects described the essential structure of caring around the following carative factors: "establishment of a human care relationship and provision of a supportive, protective, and/or corrective psychological, physical, and spiritual environment" (p. 377).

Wolf, Giardino, Osborne, and Ambrose (1994) explored the dimensions of nurse caring among nurses (278) and present and former patients (263). They used Watson's transpersonal caring theory to guide the study. From their research with these 541 subjects, using a 43-item Caring Behaviors Inventory (CBI) developed by Wolf, they conducted factor analysis to examine the conceptual fit between the items and each factor on the CBI. Five dimensions of the CBI emerged: (a) respectful deference to the other; (b) assurance of human presence; (c) positive connectedness; (d) professional knowledge and skill; and (e) attentiveness to the other's experience.

In reviewing their findings, these authors concluded:

Five factors suggest a fit of the dimensions of nurse caring with Watson's Transpersonal Theory in that nurse caring exists in consciousness. For example, the dimensions of assurance of human presence, positive connectedness, and attentiveness to the other's experience reflect the transcendent aspects of nurse caring. These factors are consistent with the perspective that caring-healing consciousness is contained in a single caring moment, takes place between the nurse and the patient, and exists through time. (1994, p. 110)

Acknowledging some limitations to their study, Wolf et al. also noted that their findings may complement other findings generated from interpretive studies on nurse caring. They concluded that these "dimensions of nurse caring could provide a framework for nurses to understand caring situations and increase their awareness of nurse and patient caring moments" (p. 111).

Harrison (1988) developed and refined a caring behaviors assessment tool based on Watson's theory of caring, using the carative factors as a framework. Cronin and Harrison (1988) used this tool as a basis for their research on caring behaviors as perceived by patients after myocardial infarction. They found that these patients identified technical behaviors related to competency as important to their caring. The instrument they developed has been used for other exploratory clinical studies in this area.

Swanson (1991) confirmed the empirical validation of Watson's theory (along with Benner's), based on her series of phenomenological studies in perinatal situations. Swanson's research generated a middle-range theory of caring, which provided a basis for conceptual cross-validation of the caring processes (Knowing, Being with, Doing for, Enabling, and Maintaining Belief) with Watson's carative factors and Benner's helping role of the nurse. Swanson reported: "The factors and role dimensions are nursing acts that universally cut across client health conditions and developmental levels. The theory of caring, carative factors, and helping role provide cross-validation for each other" (p. 165).

Swanson concluded that her own original scholarship provided a broader context for why the carative factors (and helping role) may be nurturing or helpful. Further, she noted that the convergence of these three works in her own research "supports the claim that caring is a central and unifying nursing phenomenon; it does not, however, render the concept of caring as unique to nursing knowledge or practice" (p. 165). Finally, she acknowledged that the caring theory works need to be examined in other diverse settings, including non-nursing contexts.

Ekebergh and Dahlberg (1995), working in Sweden, described the development of a caring documentation instrument (CDI) from a human caring science perspective. They identified Watson's work, along with others', as a basis for developing a documentation framework for caring. As part of their project, they implemented and evaluated a caring documentation process in a general hospital in Sweden. Their evaluation showed that the revised CDI "worked well . . .; was well-arranged . . . easy to use. The content . . . related . . . to the patients' physical health" (p. 12). While the documentation was found to be effective in some areas and began to be used, the content "was more of medical nature and the caring was missing, in several journals." This was most obvious "when the documented caring consisted of only medical measures" (p. 13). They reported that the process is an ongoing and demanding task, but recommended that the project be kept alive and continuously evaluated.

Recently, Watson's work was also used as the basis for an action research project on a transplant unit in a large teaching hospital in Sweden. The project (Watson, Sjostrom, & Gustafson, 1995) involved a form of cooperative inquiry among practicing nurses, educators, and patients at different phases of the transplant program. The caring needs and experiences of the transplant patients were related to the existential themes of "the wait, the wonder, and the watch." The nurses' caring included "responding to the presenting physical/existential concerns during each phase of the transplant experience." The transplant nurses' caring process was reported to be consistent with the caring theory; it guided the nurses' ability to be present to the patients' concerns, while also monitoring, assessing, and anticipating changes. On the basis of this study, transplant care nursing was described as "being present to, and co-participating in, the transplant patient's physical and existential experiences and caring needs, related to the trajectory of THE WAIT, THE WONDER, AND THE WATCH."

Colorado Center for Human Caring, and Its International Affiliates.   The best exemplar with respect to activities related to Watson's caring theory, both generally and specifically, is the University of Colorado Center for Human Caring, which was founded in 1986 at the University of Colorado Health Sciences Center, in the School of Nursing. The first facility of its kind, it was originally designed as an interdisciplinary, experimental think tank for the discipline of nursing. It has hosted a series of public and professional programs, sponsors in-residence faculty from nursing and other disciplines, and receives hundreds of nurses from around the world, who visit and study in the Center for short-term or year-long programs.

The Center has engaged in exploring new ways to advance the art and science of human caring; some of the efforts, conceptualized as "ontological design projects," have ranged from specific curricular activities (piloting new courses in traditional programs, for example) to initiating and supporting new educational, research, and practice (praxis) models.

Among educators, administrators, practitioners, and researchers, the Center has encouraged special initiatives that foster epistemological, ontological, methodological, and praxis inquiries associated with new ways of knowing, being, doing, practicing, and teaching caring in nursing.

Some of the published information about the Center includes the following (Watson, 1988a):

> *Formal faculty associates in the Center are exploring such areas as the moral and philosophical basis of caring, caring ethics, role of arts and humanities in a caring curriculum, and teaching and practice of caring.*
>
> *The Center also fosters nontraditional, contextual, interpretative methodological inquiries through approaches such as hermeneutics, phenomenology, literary analysis, writing (narrative-poetry), philosophical inquiry, and so on. Traditional empirical pursuits or methodologically "pragmatic" combinations are also fostered, in addition to methods that explore the "shared humanness" of caring and healing (processes and relationships), and the ontological interconnections between human [and] human, between humans and nature, and wider fields of connectedness, whether human or nonhuman.*
>
> *Consistent with the nature of caring knowledge, the Center for Human Caring advocates an interdisciplinary approach to the study and teaching of human caring; it draws directly upon the underdeveloped connections between and among the humanities and human caring-healing practices, while not neglecting traditional biomedical knowledge and practices. Collaborative interdisciplinary programs between and among other academic units on the Health Sciences Center [campus] and other campuses in the university are ongoing.*

Recently, the Center established formal International Affiliates for shared activities in other parts of the world. At the time of this writing, they include: Scottish Highlands Center for Human Caring, in the United Kingdom, headed by Dr. Elizabeth Farmer; Baycrest Gerontology Center, in Ontario, Canada, headed by Eileen Cappell (discussed earlier); Collaborative Nursing Education Project, in Victoria, British Columbia, Canada, headed by Dr. Marcia Hills; Victoria University Department of Graduate Nursing and Midwifery, Wellington, New Zealand, headed by Ms. Jill White. In addition to these formal affiliates, the Center is engaged in ongoing collaborative, consultative programs with nursing scholars at health care and academic sites in England, Portugal, Korea, Brazil, Japan, Australia, and Sweden.

All of these international (and domestic) activities are engaged in programs of study, practice, education, and research that adhere to caring as an ontological and theoretical-philosophical framework for developing the discipline and profession of nursing. Nursing caring-theory-based activities are increasing around the United States and throughout other parts of the world; Watson's work is consistently one of the nursing caring theories used as a guide. Nurses' reflective-critical practice models are invariably guided by a philosophical and theoretical nursing perspective that considers caring as a foundational ontology, even when the approach is not named ontological per se.

Most recently, the Center has developed a core curriculum in caring-healing praxis, which leads to a formal certificate. This curriculum is a professional development program for educators, clinicians, and administrators. The courses can be taken either for-credit or not-for-credit. This interdisciplinary curriculum has increasingly been taught by a combination of nurses and other health professionals, including physicians and medical scientists, whose approach is compatible with the caring-healing paradigm. The Center offers in-residence short- and long-term study programs, and sponsors Visiting Fellows and Scholars from the United States and abroad.

Information regarding the Center and its activities of study and consultation can be obtained by contacting:

Karen Holland, Executive Director
Center for Human Caring
University of Colorado Health Sciences Center
Denver, Colorado 80262
Phone: (303) 270-4331
Fax: (303) 270-8660

REFERENCES

Aucoin-Gallant, G. (1990). La thèorie du caring de Watson. Une approache existentielle-phenomologique et spirituelle des soins infirmiers. *Canadian Nurse, 86*(11), 32–35.

Bevis, E., & Watson, J. (1989). *Toward a caring curriculum: A new pedagogy for nursing*. New York: National League for Nursing.

Burns, P. (1991). Elements of spirituality and Watson's theory of transpersonal caring: Expansion of focus. In P. Chinn (Ed.), *Anthology on caring* (pp. 141-153). New York: National League for Nursing.

Cappell, E. (1994). A step-by-step guide on how to implement caring theory. In J. Watson (Ed.), *Applying the art and science of human caring*. New York: NLN Press.

Clayton, G. (1989). Research testing Watson's theory. The phenomena of caring in an elderly population. In J. Riehl-Siska (Ed.), *Conceptual models for nursing practice* (pp. 245-252). Norwalk, CT: Appleton & Lange.

Cronin, S., & Harrison, B. (1988). Importance of nurse caring behaviors as perceived by patients after myocardial infarction. *Heart & Lung, 17*(4), 374-380.

Duffy, J. (1990). *The relationship between nurse caring behaviors and selected outcomes of care in hospitalized medical and/or surgical patients*. PhD dissertation, Catholic University of America, Washington, DC.

Duffy, J. (1992). The impact of nurse caring on patient outcomes. In D. Gaut (Ed.), *The presence of caring in nursing* (pp. 113-136). New York: National League for Nursing.

Ekebergh, M., & Dahlberg, K. (1995, May). Developing a caring documentation instrument from a human caring science perspective. Paper presented at 20th International Caring Conference, Charlottesville, VA.

Fawcett, J. (1993). Watson's theory of human caring. In *Analysis and evaluation of nursing theories*. Philadelphia: Davis.

Gadow, S. (1980). Existential advocacy: Philosophical foundation of nursing. In S. Spicker & S. Gadow (Eds.), *Nursing images and ideals*. New York: Springer.

Gadow, S. (1984). Existential advocacy as a form of caring: Technology, truth, and touch. In *Research Seminar Series: The Development of Nursing as a Human Science*. Denver, CO: School of Nursing, University of Colorado Health Sciences Center.

Harrison, B. (1988). Development of the caring behaviors assessment based on Watson's theory of caring. *Master's Abstracts International, 27*, 95.

Johns, C. (Ed.). (1994). *The Burford nursing development unit model. Caring in practice*. Oxford, England: Blackwell Science.

Leininger, M. (Ed.). (1981). *Caring: An essential human need*. Thorofare, NJ: Charles B. Slack.

Leininger, M., & Watson, J. (Eds.). (1990). *The caring imperative in education*. New York: National League for Nursing.

Lemmer, C. (1991). Parental perceptions of caring following perinatal bereavement. *Western Journal of Nursing Research, 13*(4), 475–493.

McNamara, S. (1995). Perioperative nurses' perceptions of caring practices. *AORN, 61*(2), 377–388.

Pearson, A. (1983). *The clinical nursing unit*. London: Heinmann Medical Books.

Pew-Fetzer Task Force Report. (1994). *Relationship-centered care*. San Francisco: Pew Health Commission.

Sakalys, J., & Watson, J. (1985). New directions in higher education: A review of trends . . . six significant and influential reports. *Journal of Professional Nursing, 1*(5), 293–299.

Sakalys, J., & Watson, J. (1986). Professional education: Postbaccalaureate education for professional nursing . . . reintegration of the classical liberal arts model. *Journal of Professional Nursing, 2*(2), 91–97.

Schindel-Martin, L. J. (1990). A phenomenological study of faith–hope in aging clients undergoing long-term hemodialysis. *Masters Abstracts International, 28*, 583.

Schindel-Martin, L. J. (1991). Using Watson's theory to explore the dimensions of adult polycystic kidney disease. *American Nephrology Nurses' Association Journal, 18*, 493–496.

Sithichoke-Rattan, N. (1989). A clinical application of Watson's theory. *Pediatric Nursing, 15*(5), 458–462.

Swanson, K. (1991). Empirical development of a middle-range theory of caring. *Nursing Research, 40*(3), 161–166.

Teilhard de Chardin, T. (1967). *On love*. New York: Harper & Row.

Watson, J. (1985). *Nursing: The philosophy and science of caring*. Boulder, CO: Colorado Associated University Press. Original work published 1979.

Watson, J. (Ed.). (1987). *The dream curriculum*. New York: Author.

Watson, J. (1988a). A case study: Curriculum in transition. In National League for Nursing (Eds.), *Curriculum revolution: Mandate for change* (pp. 1–8). New York: National League for Nursing.

Watson, J. (1988b). Human caring as a moral context for nursing education. *Nursing and Health Care, 9*(8), 422–425.

Watson, J. (1988c). *Nursing: Human science and human care: A theory of nursing*. New York: National League for Nursing. Original work published 1985.

Watson, J. (1988d). The professional doctorate as an entry level into practice: Based on presentations at the eighteenth NLN biennial convention. In National League for Nursing (Eds.), *Perspective in nursing: 1987-1989* (pp. 41-48). New York: National League for Nursing.

Watson, J. (1989). Keynote address: Caring theory. *Journal of Japan Academy of Nursing Science, 9*(2), 29-37.

Watson, J. (1990). Transformation in nursing: Bringing care back to health care. In E. Bevis & J. Watson (Eds.), *Toward a caring curriculum: A new pedagogy for nursing* (pp. 15-20). New York: National League for Nursing.

Watson, J., & Bevis, E. (1990). Nursing education: Coming of age for a new age. In N. L. Chaska (Eds.), *The nursing profession, turning points* (pp. 100-106). St. Louis: C. V. Mosby.

Watson, J., Sjostrom, B., & Gustafson, M. (1995). Research in Brief 49: The wait, the wonder, the watch: Caring in a transplant unit. *Journal of Clinical Nursing.*

Wolf, Z., Giardino, E., Osborne, P., & Ambrose, M. S. (1994). Dimensions of nurse caring. *Image: The Journal of Nursing Scholarship, 26*(2), 107-111.

Zukav, G. (1990). *The seat of the soul.* New York: Fireside Books.

Section IV

Blueprints for Practice

7

Levine's Conservation Model: Caring for Women with Chronic Illness

Karen Moore Schaefer

Over the past eight years, Myra Levine critiqued, supported, and encouraged my use of the Conservation Model. Perhaps most important, she encouraged my creative applications of the model. I shared the following chapter with her, hoping that once again she would respond constructively to my use and inter- pretation of the model. She "felt a little empty on [my] discussion of health" (Levine, personal communication, February 21, 1995) and went on to say ". . . it is not an entity, but rather a definition imparted by the ethos and be- liefs of the groups to which the individual belongs." Inspired by her critique, I modified portions of the chapter to reflect her beliefs about health in the care of women with chronic illness. Health may be difficult to define, both globally and individually, but use of the Conservation Model assists the nurse with the development of an approach to care that will attend to the individual needs and desires of women with chronic illness. As we move into the 21st century

*and we experience an increase in the number of women living with chronic ill-
nesses, advanced practice nurses are encouraged to expand the use of the Conservation Model by integrating adjunctive theories and models to support
integrative health care delivery and to facilitate the transitions in new models
of care. "This chapter is dedicated to Myra Levine who passed away on
March 20, 1996. We have lost a visionary nursing leader: I have lost a dear
friend and colleague. Her encouragement, support, honesty and candid critique will be missed!"*

Karen Moore Schaefer

BRIEF DESCRIPTION OF THE MODEL

Over the years, I have come to realize that my practice, research,
and teaching experiences are all part of my unique expression of
nursing as human interaction. For the past ten years, the majority of
my research has focused on chronic illness in women. While learning about women's experiences with chronic illness, I have been introducing graduate students to Myra Levine's Conservation Model
and encouraging use of the model as a framework for research in
areas such as sleep disturbances and fatigue. Subsequently, use of
the model has become a natural part of my thinking as a professional nurse.

As part of my research, I have been privileged to serve as a consultant and speaker for support groups of women with chronic fatigue syndrome and fibromyalgia (FM). My discussions with the
women attending the support groups are understood and embraced
more readily when I use the Conservation Model as a framework.
The women express a continued need to learn to manage *life with
the illness* and to feel "normal" again. Levine, understanding this
need, states that "even when the disease process cannot be elimi-
nated and a new life style must be developed, well-being (wholeness) continues to be a goal" (Levine, 1971a, p. 9).

When used in practice, Levine's Conservation Model provides
nurses with a framework through which to view individuals as
holistic, active, and self-determining. The goals of promoting adaptation and maintaining wholeness are consistent with the desired

outcomes of women with chronic illness. The model also values patients' participation in the planning of care, and the women value having a role in setting up their health care regimen. The model provides a logical and practical way to discuss their experiences and to explore the interventions that can help them achieve comfort in living with their illness. Responses to interventions are always evaluated at the organismic level, keeping the women at the center of the experience.

PHILOSOPHICAL BASIS OF THE MODEL

Theoretical Background

Levine's Conservation Model incorporates knowledge from the physical, social, psychological, and biological sciences. Levine draws from her personal experiences as a nurse and as a patient (personal communication, May 17, 1989). Levine (1973a) credits Bernard (1957), Waddington (1968), Goldstein (1963), Gibson (1966), Dubos (1965), Bates (1967), Hall (1966), Erickson (1968), Beland (1971), and Wolf (1961) as scholars who influenced her work.

Bernard (1957) is acknowledged for his identification of the interdependence of bodily functions in the *milieu interne* (internal environment) (Levine, 1973a). Using Waddington's (1968) term *homeorhesis,* Levine emphasized the dynamic nature of the *milieu interne.* Her discussion of homeorhesis clarifies that individuals are organismic rather than mechanistic in nature. Human beings seek stability when challenged by factors in their external environment, but the outcome is dynamic rather than static. Conceptually, individuals are in a constant state of dynamic interaction.

Levine (1973a) rejected a simplistic view of the environment and adopted Bates's (1967) formulation of the external environment as a perceptual, operational, and conceptual source of factors that provide ongoing challenges to the integrity of the individual. She based her description of illness on Wolf's (1961) description of disease as adaptation to noxious environmental forces. She believes that, although illness challenges individual integrity, defending one's health is an ongoing endeavor (Levine, 1991).

Levine (1989c) incorporated Selye's (1956) definition of stress in her description of the organismic stress response as being "recorded over time and . . . influenced by the accumulated experience of the individual" (p. 30). Gibson's (1966) work on perception as a mediator of behavior and his classification of the five perceptual systems contributed to Levine's development of the perceptual organismic response of the individual in interaction with the environment. The five perceptual systems included in the response are hearing (balancing portion of the inner ear), sight (visual system), touch (haptic system), taste, and smell. Levine notes that individuals are defined by information received through intact and functional perceptual systems.

Goldstein's (1963) description of brain-injured soldiers who, despite severe disability, sought to cling to some semblance of self-awareness provided support for Levine's (1973a, 1991) belief that individuals seek to defend their personhood. The process of change seeks "congruence" (Goldstein, 1963) with the environment. Levine references DuBos's (1965) discussion of the adaptability of organisms to support her premise that similarities of adaptation exist within a wide range of responses (Levine, 1989c). Nightingale (1859) is credited by Levine (1992) for providing a basis for her concept of observation as a "guardian activity" of nursing that is used to "save lives and increase health and comfort" (p. 41), Levine reemphasizes Nightingale's use of conservation principles in her work. In particular, Levine links her discussion of social integrity to Nightingale's concern for sanitation, implying that the environment—including social, political, and cultural factors—and the individual continually interact.

As a patient, Levine (personal communication, May 17, 1989) experienced firsthand how ill persons seek to defend their integrity, their wholeness (health). Through a difficult challenge from both her external and internal environment, she reinforced her belief in the importance of the conservation principles. Her experience was very complex, involving energy imbalance along with metabolic and genetic level changes. In dealing with this very difficult insult, it was important that the nurses helped conserve her dignity, as well as her strength, throughout the ordeal. She concluded that "every self-sustaining system monitors its own behavior by conserving the use of resources it needs to define its unique identity."

Purpose of the Model

The Conservation Model, as an organizing framework for nursing practice, promotes adaptation and maintains wholeness using the principle of conservation. It guides the nurse to focus on the influences and responses at the organismic level (Dever, 1991). The nurse accomplishes the model's goals through the conservation of energy and of structural, personal, and social integrity simultaneously (Foreman, 1991; Schaefer, 1990; Schaefer & Potylycki, 1993). Interventions are either supportive or therapeutic; outcomes are assessed through the observation of organismic responses.

Concepts

Levine identifies two major concepts in her model: (1) adaptation and (2) wholeness. Conservation, a fundamental principle of the model, is addressed as the outcome of adaptation.

Adaptation. Adaptation is the ongoing process of change—the life process—whereby individuals retain their integrity within the reality of their environment (Levine, 1989c). Adaptation, the method of change, is achieved by ". . . the frugal, economic, contained, and controlled use of environmental resources by the individual in his or her best interest" (Levine, 1991, p. 5). Levine states further that:

> . . . *The environmental "fit" that underscores successful adaptation suggests that every species has fixed patterns of response uniquely designed to ensure success in essential life activities, demonstrating that adaptation is both historical and specific. However, tremendous opportunities for individual accommodations are locked into the gene structure of each species; every individual is one of a kind. (p. 5)*

Every individual possesses a unique range of adaptive responses. A person's ranges may vary with age or when challenged by illness. This variation is evidenced when the hypoxic drive provides the stimulus for breathing in individuals with chronic obstructive pulmonary disease.

Adaptations, characterized by redundancy, history, and specificity, are "rooted in history and waiting the specific circumstances to which they respond" (Levine, 1991, p. 6). The genetic structure, developed over time, provides the foundation for a range of adaptive responses. Specificity, while sharing traits with a species, has individual potential, and this potential creates the variety of adaptational goals (Levine, 1989). For example, there is some speculation that fibromyalgia may be genetic because it "seems to run in families." The severity of response and the adaptive patterns of women with FM will vary, based on the specific genetic structure and the influence of social, cultural, and experiential factors.

Redundancy represents the fail-safe anatomical, physiological, and psychological options available to the individual to ensure continued adaptation. "Achieving health is predicated on the deliberate selection of redundant options" (Levine, 1991, p. 6). Survival is dependent on these redundant options, which are challenged and often limited by illness, disease, and aging. For example, when one kidney is transplanted into another individual, the remaining kidney continues the work of the original two kidneys. When options are no longer available, survival becomes difficult. Adaptation thus represents accommodation between the internal and external environments.

Conservation is the product of adaptation. Conservation is a universal principle, a natural law, that is common to many of the basic sciences (Levine, 1991). In the Victorian era, when Nightingale was a young girl, conservation was fundamental to Mitchell's Rest Cure for the common female malady, hysteria (Ehrenreich & English, 1992). Conserving energy was necessary for healing to take place, but modern feminists claim the cure was simply another way in which women were oppressed by the reigning male physicians of the era. Women were not permitted to have a voice, and the rest cure only perpetuated their voiceless status by not permitting the women to write or have visitors.

Conservation of energy, according to Levine, is very different from the mechanistic rest cure intervention of the Victorian era. Identification of conservation's universal importance makes it an essential element in understanding human life. Levine (1991) says:

> *Implicit in the knowledge of conservation in the fact of wholeness, integrity, unity—all of the structures that are* being conserved. . . . *conservation of the integrity of the person is essential to ensuring health and providing the strength to confront disability. . . . the importance of conservation is the treatment of illness is precisely*

focused on the reclamation of wholeness, of health. . . . Every nursing act is dedicated to the conservation, or "keeping together," of the wholeness of the individual. (p. 3)

Individuals are continuously defending their wholeness. Conservation is the *keeping together* of the life system. Individuals defend that system in constant interaction with their environment, choosing the most economical, frugal, energy-sparing options available to safeguard their integrity. Conservation aims to achieve a balance of energy supply and demand that is within the unique biological capacities of the individual.

To *keep together* means to maintain a proper balance between active nursing interventions coupled with patient participation, on the one hand, and the safe limits of a patient's ability to participate, on the other. An energy source cannot be directly observed, but the consequences (clinical manifestations) of its exchange are predictable, manageable, and recognizable (Levine, 1991).

Wholeness. Levine (1973a) bases her interpretation of wholeness on Erickson's (1968) description of wholeness as an open system: "Wholeness emphasizes a sound, organic, progressive mutuality between diversified functions and parts within an entirety, the boundaries of which are open and fluid" (p. 93). Levine states that "the unceasing interaction of the individual organism with its environment does represent an 'open and fluid' system, and a condition of health, or wholeness, exists when the interactions, or constant adaptations to the environment, permit ease—the assurance of integrity . . . in all the dimensions of life" (1973a, p. 11). Recognition of an open, fluid, constantly changing interaction between the individual and the environment is the basis for holistic thought, the view of the individual as a whole.

Women with fibromyalgia describe the process of living with their illness as one of adapting to a level of function that is acceptable to them. They emphasize that adaptation is a continuous process that does not imply or mean the same as *acceptance.* Most women suggest that *acceptance* means resignation to the illness, which can be equated with *giving in* and not actively seeking wellness.

Their frustrations with the traditional health care system are attributed to physicians who do not recognize their concerns as valid and who are unable to treat them as whole individuals. Their complaints are interpreted as disease, and when disease cannot be validated, the women believe they are viewed by the physicians as unreliable, invisible, neurotic, and highly stressed. They seek acceptance as persons with valid experiences of illness that continuously challenge their integrity. They seek assistance in managing their illness when they are no longer able to do so on their own.

Subconcepts (Commonplaces)

Subconcepts or commonplaces of the Conservation Model include person, nursing, health, and environment. Levine (1988) calls them *commonplaces of the discipline* because they are necessary for any description of nursing.

Person. The person is a holistic being who is sentient, thinking, future-oriented, and past-aware. The wholeness (integrity) of the individual demands that the "isolated aspects . . . can have meaning outside of the context within which the individual experiences his or her life . . ." (Levine, 1973a, pp. 325–326). Persons are in constant interaction with the environment; they respond to change in an orderly, sequential pattern. They are thus adapting to forces that shape and reshape the essence of the person. According to Levine, the person can be defined as an individual, an individual in a group (family), or an individual in a community (Pond, 1991).

Environment. The environment completes the wholeness of the person. Each individual is viewed as having his or her own internal and external environment. The internal environment, which combines the physiological and pathophysiological aspects of the patient, is constantly challenged by changes in the external environment.

The external environment includes those factors that impinge on and challenge the individual. Acknowledging the complexity of the environment, Levine (1973a) adopted the three levels of environment identified by Bates (1967). The *perceptual* environment includes aspects of the world that individuals are able to intercept or interpret through the senses. Levine (1971a) states, "The individual is not a passive recipient of sensory input . . . [but] seeks, selects, and tests information from the environment in the context of his [her] definition of himself [herself], and so defends his [her] safety, his [her] identity, and in a larger sense, his [her] purpose" (p. 262).

The *operational* environment includes elements that may physically affect individuals but are not directly perceived by them, such as radiation and micro-organisms. The *conceptual* environment includes the cultural patterns characterized by spiritual existence and mediated by symbols of language, thought, and history. Factors that affect behavior, such as values and beliefs, are part of the conceptual environment.

Health.   Health and disease are patterns of adaptive change, one of the goals of which is well-being (Levine, 1971b). Health from a social perspective is defined in the question: "Do I continue to function in a reasonably normal fashion?" (Levine, 1984). A definition of health (wholeness) as the unity and integrity of the individual is implied. Health (wholeness) is the goal of nursing. Levine (1991) says:

> *Health is the avenue of return to the daily activities compromised by ill health. It is not only the insult or the injury that is repaired but the person himself or herself.... It is not merely the healing of an afflicted part. It is rather a return to selfhood, where the encroachment of the disability can be set aside entirely, and the individual is free to pursue once more his or her own interests without constraint. (p. 4)*

She further stresses, "It is important to keep in mind that health is also [sic] culturally determined—it is not an entity on its own, but rather a definition imparted by the ethos and beliefs of the groups to which individuals belong" (Levine, personal communication, February 21, 1995). Even for a single individual, what is identified as health may change over time, affected by new situations, new life, age, or social, political, economic, and spiritual factors. In all life challenges, individuals will always attempt to regain, sustain, or protect their health (wholeness).

Illness is described as adaptation to noxious environmental forces. "Disease represents the individual's effort to protect self integrity, such as the inflammatory system's response to injury" (Levine, 1971a, p. 257). Disease is unregulated and undisciplined change; it must be stopped, or death will ensue (Levine, 1973a).

Nursing.   Nursing is an art and a science (Levine, 1988). Nurses engage in "human interaction" (Levine, 1973a, p. 1). "The nurse enters into a partnership of human experience where sharing moments in time—some trivial, some dramatic—leaves its mark forever on each patient" (Levine, 1977, p. 845). The goal of nursing is to promote adaptation and maintain wholeness (health). This goal is accomplished through the conservation of energy, structure, person, and social integrity.

Energy conservation is dependent on free energy exchange with the environment, so that living systems can constantly replenish their energy supply (Levine, 1991). Conservation of energy is integral to the individual's range of adaptive responses. The conservation of structural integrity is dependent on an intact defense system that supports repair and healing and that is responsive to the challenges from the internal and external environments.

The conservation of personal integrity recognizes the individual who establishes his or her wholeness in response to the environment. It acknowledges that individuals strive for recognition, respect, self-awareness, humanness, selfhood, and self-determination.

Conservation of social integrity recognizes that individuals function in a society that helps to establish the boundaries of the self. It acknowledges that persons are valued for their individuality but also have the need to belong to a family, a community, a religious group, an ethnic group, a political system, and a nation (Levine, 1973a). "Conservation of integrity is essential to assuring wholeness [sic] and providing the strength needed [sic] to confront illness [sic] and disability" (Levine, 1991, p. 3).

Nurses use the scientific process to make observations and select relevant data that allow forming hypothetical statements about the patients' predicaments (Schaefer, 1991). According to Levine (1966b), this scientific process is called "trophicognosis" (p. 57). Use of the scientific process assumes that the nurse encounters the patients' experience with the knowledge base necessary to make statements (judgments). This knowledge base gives the provocative facts meaning. Using the provocative facts, the nurse establishes a hypothesis that will direct the nursing interventions. In essence, the hypothesis is being tested. The nurse observes, seeking an organismic response. If the patient responds, the hypothesis is supported. If the patient does not respond, the hypothesis is not supported, and the nurse reexamines the provocative facts and reformulates the hypothesis.

Relationships Among the Concepts and Subconcepts

Conservation, adaptation, and well-being are linked in the following statement: "Survival depends on the adaptive ability to use responses that cost the least to the individual in expense of effort and demand on his or her well-being" (Levine, 1989c, p. 329).

Linkages of all four subconcepts (commonplaces) are made in the following statements:

> *The nurse participates actively in every patient's environment, and much of what she does supports his adaptations as he struggles in the predicament of illness. (Levine, 1973a, p. 13)*

> *But even in the presence of disease, the organism responds wholly to the environmental interaction in which it is involved, and a considerable element of nursing care is devoted to restoring the symmetry of response—symmetry that is essential to the well-being of the organism. (Levine, 1969b, p. 98)*

The subconcepts defined within the Conservation Model fit the experience of women with chronic illness (fibromyalgia). Their ability to live with the illness depends a great deal on the availability of alternative approaches to care. Research suggests that women diagnosed with the disorder respond in an unique yet similar fashion (Schaefer, 1995a). The unique experiences emphasize the validity and specificity of adaptation and the importance of redundant options for survival, options from which individuals can select approaches that assist them in achieving a sense of well-being. They frequently measure their success based on their ability to maintain balance in life. Their goal is to feel as whole as possible. Every conservation, ability to function, feeling good about themselves, and being able to engage in social activities, including gainful employment, are important to their personhood.

For nurses to help women with chronic illness achieve their goals, they must exercise their voices relative to the social and political factors in the external environment that impact the health and well-being of these women. The Conservation Model provides a framework for these activities. Attention to the conceptual environment focuses the nurse on the environmental factors that are perceived as challenging to the individual. These factors include an

understanding of the historical roots of women's health care, the social factors that perpetuate a minimal social value for the work of
women, the cultural and religious factors that influence behavior,
and the political and social factors that keep the women "barefoot
and dumb" (Inlander, 1992). Little is known about the structural integrity of the women because the syndrome has been dismissed as
psychological. Women and nurses must continue to support efforts
that allocate research moneys to find a cause of this sometimes disabling syndrome.

Structure of the Model

The structure of the model encourages the nurse to use all available
health care information and research to establish the basis for a
nursing plan of care for individuals who are no longer able to adapt
on their own. These individuals are appropriately called patients because they are in a temporary predicament of suffering that allows
them to "set aside independence and accept the services of another"
(Levine, 1989a, p. 126). Patients are "individuals with strengths and
individuality, certain of their selfhood, unique, proud, and more
than just a target that will respond" (Levine, 1987, p. 50). They accept their patient status not as passive recipients of care but like Job
who "argued, complained, lamented and despised his underserved
misfortune" (Levine, 1989a, p. 126).

Levine (1973a) makes explicit the importance of understanding
the medical plan of care and the results of diagnostic studies to an
accurate understanding of patient problems. To this understanding,
the nurse brings knowledge of nursing science, a careful history of
the patient's illness, the patient's perception of the current predicament, information gained from family and friends, and acute observation of the patient and his or her interactions with others (Levine,
1966a). This integrated approach to patient-centered care provides
the basis for collaborative care or the establishment of partnerships
in the delivery of comprehensive care. Levine (1987) charges us to
join forces with our colleagues to "explore clinical issues that we
must confront together" (p. 51).

The nature of chronic illness betrays the most sophisticated
medical research. Chronicity implies *no cause, no cure.* Treatment

focuses on the management of the organismic responses to the illness. Levine (1971b) says that "the study of individuals in sickness and health demonstrates that every response involves the entire individual in some degree" (p. 6). This organismic response emphasizes that "every aspect of the organism is involved in all of its interactions with its environment" (Levine, 1971b, p. 6). Organismic responses include flight/fight response, immune system response, stress response, and perceptual awareness. Flight/fight, the most primitive response, sets up physiological and behavioral readiness to cope with or withdraw from a real or imagined threat. The inflammatory/immune system provides for structural continuity and promotion of healing, and the stress response is recorded over time and is influenced by the accumulated experience of the individual. Prolonged stress can lead to damage within these systems. The perceptual response involves gathering information from the environment and converting it to a meaningful experience. These four responses work together to protect the individual's integrity. The physiological and behavioral responses are essential components of the individual's whole response.

The goal of nursing care is to promote adaptation and well-being. Because adaptation is predicated on redundant options and rooted in history and specificity, therapeutic interventions will vary, based on the unique nature of each person's response. This is repeatedly demonstrated by the wide range in insulin dosages among individuals with diabetes, as well as the types of insulin used in treatment. Equally relevant is the observation that, although a specific intervention may work for one women with FM, it may not work for another. The goal of the nurse is to recognize the individuality of each person.

The individual's internal and external environments are given careful attention in order to locate sources of compromise. Challenges in the internal environment of women with FM are poorly understood, but they include the possibility of lack of stage IV sleep, disturbance in hormone function, and changes in immune system function. Challenges in the external environment include factors such as changing weather conditions (Schaefer, 1995), toxic chemicals (hair spray, smoke), and abandonment by health professionals, coworkers, and friends. Organismic responses include aches, pain, fatigue, sleeplessness, weakness, stomach upset, headaches, depression, anger, and anxiety.

The nurse is responsible for recognizing this state of altered health and the patient's unique organismic response to altered health. The nurse observes the patient: "Observation means to guard against and is then a guardian angel. . . . A guardian angel suggests an assumption of responsibility and concern based on the knowledge that makes it possible to decide in the patient's behalf and in his [her] best interests" (Levine, 1971b, p. 17).

Once the organismic responses are identified, the nurse establishes a hypothetical statement about the problem and designs interventions that will support or refute the original hypothesis. According to Levine, interventions are either therapeutic or supportive. Therapeutic interventions are those interventions that influence adaptation favorably or help create new social well-being (Levine, 1973a). Supportive nursing interventions are provided when the outcome cannot be changed; the goals are comfort and maintenance of the status quo. For example, the aches and pains that women with FM experience are proposed to be the result of a lack of restful sleep (stage IV sleep). Nursing research (Lentz, Shaver, & Heitkemper, 1993) suggests that rather than changes in the alpha waves, there is a reduction in the delta waves. If this is the case, interventions that will increase the body temperature, subsequently increasing the delta waves, should change the organismic response. Taking a warm bath before retiring may improve the quality of sleep. If the patient reports restful sleep and a reduction in pain intensity, the hypothesis is supported. There has been no cure, but the intervention is therapeutic because it has changed the organismic response.

The structure of the model provides the basis for two developing theories for practice: (a) the Theory of Therapeutic Intention and (b) the Theory of Redundancy. In developing the Theory of Therapeutic Intention, Levine (cited in Fawcett, 1995) was "seeking a way of organizing nursing interventions out of the biological realities which the nurse had to confront" (p. 198). Therapeutic regimens should support the following goals:

1. Facilitate integrated healing and optimal restoration of structure and function through natural response to disease.

2. Provide support for a failing autoregulatory portion of the integrated system (medical/surgical treatments).

3. Restore individual integrity and well-being.

4. Provide supportive measures to ensure comfort and promote human concern when therapeutic measures are not possible.

5. Balance a toxic risk against the threat of disease.

6. Manipulate diet and activity to correct metabolic imbalances and stimulate physiological processes.

7. Reinforce or antagonize the usual response to create a therapeutic change. (cited in Fawcett, 1995)

Levine (1978, cited in Fawcett, 1995) proposed that the Theory of Redundancy, seemingly grounded in adaptation, "redefines almost everything that has to do with human life. . . . [A]ging is the diminished availability of redundant systems necessary for effective maintenance of physical and social well-being."

Redundancy seems to be predicated on the ability of the individual to:

> . . . monitor [his or her] own behavior by conserving the use of the resources required to define [his or her] unique identity. The ability of every individual not only to survive but to flourish is a consequence of the competence of the person's interactions with the environment in which he or she functions. Every successful organism has the ability to select from the environment those elements that are essential to its welfare and to exclude those that are repetitive, harmful, or inconsequential. (Levine, 1991, pp. 4, 5)

Inherent in this ability to select from the environment is the availability of options from which choices can be made:

> . . . the ubiquitous presence of fail-safe options in the anatomy, physiology, and psychology of individuals represents a redundancy easily identified and often employed in planning health care. The choice of one strategy instead of another rests with the knowledge of the health care planner. Often there is tacit recognition that more than one solution is possible. Achieving health, as the individual experiences it, is predicated on a deliberate selection of redundant options. When the individual loses redundant

*choices as a consequence of disease, trauma, aging, or environ-
mental circumstances, survival becomes difficult and ultimately
fails for lack of fail-safe options—either those that the person possesses or those that can be employed in his or her behalf. . . .
(Levine, 1991, p. 6)*

Assumptions

The Conservation Model is based on the following assumptions:

1. Person [sic] is viewed as a holistic being. "The experience of wholeness is the foundation of all human enterprise" (Levine, 1991, p. 3).

2. "Ultimately, decisions for nursing intervention are based on the unique behavior of the individual patient. . . . A theory of nursing must recognize the importance of unique detail of care for a single patient within a empiric framework which successfully describes the requirements of all patients" (Levine, 1973a, p. 6).

3. "Patient-centered nursing care means individualized nursing care. It is predicated on the reality of common experience: every man is a unique individual, and as such he requires a unique constellation of skills, techniques, and ideas designed specially for him" (Levine, 1973a, p. 23).

4. The person can only be understood within the context of his or her environment (Levine, 1973a).

5. Every self-sustaining system monitors its own behavior by conserving the use of the resources required to define its unique identity (Levine, 1991, p. 4).

6. Human beings respond in a singular yet integrated fashion. "While the diseases that afflict man may be studied system by system or even cell by cell, the experience of life has taught repeatedly that each individual responds wholly and completely to every alteration in his life pattern" (Levine, 1971b, p. 6). Levine goes on to stress that "Recognition of the wholeness of the individual is a necessary correlate of effective nursing care; only the recognition of many kinds of responses occurring

simultaneously in a single individual offers any hope that his fundamental requirements will be met" (p. 7).

7. Finally and fundamentally, nursing is a unique contributor to patient care (Levine, 1989d).

Values

1. All nursing actions are moral actions.

2. Two moral imperatives of nursing are the sanctity of life and the relief of suffering.

3. Ethical behavior "is the day-to-day expression of one's commitment to other persons and the ways in which human beings relate to one another in their daily interactions" (Levine, 1977, p. 846).

4. Decisions regarding life and death should be made in advance of the situations by a fully informed individual (advanced directives). These decisions are not the role of health care providers or families (Levine, 1989d).

5. Judgments by nurses or doctors about quality of life are inappropriate and should not be used as a basis for the allocation of care (Levine, 1989d).

6. "Persons who require the intensive interventions of critical care units enter with a contract of trust. To respect trust . . . is a moral responsibility" (Levine, 1989d, p. 88).

PRACTICAL ASPECTS OF THE CONSERVATION MODEL

The Conservation Model was not originally developed as a model for practice; it was as an organizing framework for teaching undergraduate nursing students (Levine, 1971b). Levine's book made a significant contribution to the "whys" of nursing actions. Levine was intent on not simply teaching the skill of nursing but also providing a rationale for the behaviors. She has shown a high regard for the integration of adjunctive sciences to develop a theoretical basis of nursing (Levine, 1988), and she has continued to call attention to the rhetoric of nursing (Levine, 1989b, 1994).

The universality of the Conservation Model is supported by its use with a variety of patients of differing ages in a spectrum of settings. The model has been successfully used in critical care (Brunner, 1985; Langer, 1990; Littrell & Schumann, 1989; Lynn-McHale & Smith, 1991; Tribotti, 1990), acute care (Foreman, 1991; Molchany, 1993; Schaefer, 1991), patients in long-term care (Cox, 1991), and patients in the community (Pond, 1991). The Conservation Model has also been used with the neonate (Tribotti, 1990), the infant (Newport, 1984; Savage & Culbert, 1989), the young child (Dever, 1991), the pregnant woman (Roberts, Fleming, & Yeates-Giese, 1991), the young adult (Pasco & Halupa, 1991), and the elderly (Cox, 1991; Foreman, 1991; Hirschfeld, 1976). It has been successfully used in the community (Pond, 1991), emergency room (Pond & Taney, 1991), extended care facility (Cox, 1991), critical care unit (Brunner, 1985; Molchany, 1993), primary care clinic (Pond, 1991), and operating room (Crawford-Gamble, 1986). The model has been used as a framework for wound care (Cooper, 1990) and care of intravenous sites (Dibble, Bostrom-Exrati, & Rizzuto, 1991), and for patients undergoing treatment for cancer (O'Laughlin, 1986; Webb, 1993). Discussion about its use with the frail elderly is underway (M. Happ, personal communication, January, 31, 1995), and its application in the administrative arena is being considered (Cox, personal communication, February 21, 1995). Because of wider use of the model in hospitals and communities, nurse educators are bringing it into more and more undergraduate and graduate training, where it has been successfully integrated (Grindley & Paradowski, 1991; Schaefer, 1991).

USE OF THE MODEL IN PRACTICE: CARE OF WOMEN WITH CHRONIC ILLNESS

Understanding of the Medical Plan of Care

Fibromyalgia (FM) is a chronic painful muscle disorder that is most commonly first diagnosed in women between the ages of 20 and 45

(Rothchild, 1991). Diagnosis is made by exclusion of other disorders and a lack of any definitive physiological changes. Most diagnostic studies show no abnormality; yet the individuals feel terrible. Some may have an elevated sedimentation rate. If so, some other process is probably responsible. The symptoms (generally) mimic the flu and include muscle aches and pains, stiffness, nausea, and fatigue (Boissevain & McCain, 1991).

Research findings to date are inconclusive. There have been suggestions of physiological disturbance related to cellular hypoxia (Bennett et al., 1989), abnormal protein breakdown (Boissevain & McCain, 1991), hormonal imbalance (McCain & Tilbe, 1989), retrovirus (Martin, 1993), brain wave disturbances (Lentz, Shaver, & Heitkemper, 1993; Moldofsky, 1989), and immune system dysfunction (Daily, Bishop, Russell, & Fletcher, 1990). Sleep research findings reveal a common lack of adequate stage IV sleep (nonrestorative sleep patterns) in individuals diagnosed with FM. The most successful medical treatment for FM includes the use of amitriptyline in low doses, cyclobenzaprine, hypnotics (triazolam, alprazolam), physical therapy, and emotional support. With little success in identifying a cause, treatment is based on reported case studies and limited clinical comparisons. Clinical trials have not yet been reported. Longitudinal studies to understand the ongoing processes are still needed.

The disorder, at first, was attributed to personality style. The personality profile suggested that women who were diagnosed with FM were physically unfit, had a history of depression, were oversensitive, and were hypochondriacs (Shorter, 1992). Women reported, "I thought I was going crazy"; "They thought it was all in my head"; "My doctor told me that it had to be in my head because no symptoms traveled from one place in my body to another like mine did." This profile could not be clinically validated.

The actual diagnosis of FM, for some women, is a relief after years of fearing insanity or a series of life-threatening alternatives such as multiple sclerosis or a brain tumor. For others, the diagnosis is devastating. Initial medical treatment may alleviate the symptoms for some individuals, but others have little or no success with traditional medical therapy. Those individuals who have some initial relief eventually learn that the symptoms *break through* the treatment.

Chronic uncertainty about the natural history of the disease adds to the disabling effects. Economic, social, and political support are almost nonexistent, although recent efforts to secure funding have been successful.

Medical treatment has limited value. The disorder is probably best treated using a variety of nonpharmacological and holistic health care interventions that are less costly and more fitting to individual preferences. Women with FM need the compassion and caring that are at the center of nursing practice. There may be no known cause, but the experience is real for the patient. Nurses' goals in caring are to maintain integrity (selfhood) and promote adaptation. Recognizing the patient's difficulty in adapting, nurses provide the patient with alternative interventions that will improve the quality of life.

Developing and Implementing the Nursing Plan of Care

When Levine's Conservation Model is used as a basis of nursing practice, the focus of nursing care is on maintenance of wholeness (integrity, oneness) and promotion of adaptation. The nurse enters into a relationship with patients when their integrity is threatened and their usual self-care techniques are no longer effective or cannot be done without assistance. Levine (1973a) calls this relationship a "predicament" or a difficult situation involving choices. The situation is difficult because patients are temporarily dependent on the caring behaviors of the nurse when they would prefer to be independent. In this relationship, the nurse respects the individuals' privacy and personhood. To maintain wholeness and promote adaptation, the nurse involves the patients in the decisions about their care and provides patients with alternative approaches to care.

Entering into a Relationship

Women with FM are seen more often in the community than in the hospital. Patients with FM are generally not admitted to a hospital for treatment, but many women may have FM as a secondary or underlying diagnosis. Routine assessments often reveal that the patient has little or no understanding of the syndrome.

As the nurse and the patient enter into a relationship, the nurse encourages the patient to explain the predicament. Attention to the environmental factors and the integrities helps to ensure that the patient's sense of oneness is maintained even during an initial encounter. For patients with FM, this approach is extremely important. These patients have had some experience with rejection related to disbelief that something was really wrong. They may doubt their integrity and feel that they no longer have control over their lives. This feeling is supported by research; women are not taken seriously and their concerns are not perceived as valid (Schaefer, 1995a).

Environment

The prescribed environment completes the wholeness of the person (Levine, 1973a). Persons can be understood only within the context of the environment. Levine defines both an internal and an external environment. The individual responds to the constant interplay of the internal and external environments with an organismic response, in an attempt to adapt. Organismic responses include the response to fear, the inflammatory response, the stress response, and the sensory response, which converts energy into meaningful experiences. Adaptation represents accommodation between the external and internal environment.

Internal. Assessment typically reveals that the women have "been treating pains for years." It is not uncommon for these women to say, "The doctors did all these tests and found nothing wrong with me. All the tests were normal." They may report a history of difficult menstrual periods (PMS), frequent intestinal problems (irritable bowel), allergies, and migraine headaches. One woman said, "I always had problems with my knee and was sure I had early arthritis, but repeated X-rays found nothing." Objective data seldom support the disease (medical) model. There may be a history of slightly abnormal laboratory studies (e.g., elevated sedimentation rate, Epstein-Barr virus, elevated liver enzymes), but the present physiological and pathophysiological aspects are found to be normal.

External. Levine's external environment includes three levels adapted from the work by Bates (1967): perceptual, operational, and conceptual. The perceptual environment is the portion of the environment that the individual responds to with sense organs. The operational environment is the elements for which the person has no sense, such as micro-organisms and pollutants, but which may affect the person's behavior. Pollutants may be blamed for some of the symptoms. One woman noted that she could no longer use hair sprays or spray deodorants because she was allergic to them. Because of her allergies, she avoided paint or anything that had volatility. She claimed she felt better after being more careful, thus supporting Levine's (1991) notion that a person seeks, selects, and tests information from the environment in the context of his or her definition of self, thus defending personal safety, identity, and purpose.

The conceptual environment encompasses language, thought, emotion, values, religious beliefs, and ethnic and cultural traditions. This environment takes into account that human beings are "sentient, thinking, future-oriented and past-aware" (Levine, 1989c, p. 326). Adaptation to the conceptual environment is sometimes threatened by a response implying that the complaints associated with the illness are not valid.

Reflective thinking by women with FM often brings to mind a family member who always suffered from headaches, or who complained of legs that ached all the time. Ethnic and cultural influences are evidenced when women talk about the need to "go on" or "make do." There seems to be a tradition of doing whatever they have to do to make the best of a difficult situation. Socially, on the other hand, women are often accused of malingering, and men are viewed as stoic.

Conservation Principles

Concern for the conservation of energy—the conservation of structural, personal, and social integrity—further ensures that the women feel whole. They do not see themselves as persons made up of parts not related to the whole. Interventions that consider each principle in interaction with all other principles are more likely to maintain integrity and promote adaptation than are interventions that focus on a single principle and exclude the others.

Energy Conservation. The principle of energy conservation focuses on assessment of which activities may contribute to placing an energy drain on an actual or perceived insufficient energy supply. It is important to consider women's special energy needs during pregnancy, during menopause, in times of emotional stress, and when required to juggle work and family schedules. During pregnancy, there is a normal increase in need for rest; during the first and third trimester, that need may be more pronounced if the woman has FM. The fatigue associated with menopause may be accentuated and incorrectly interpreted as worsening FM when it may be related to a lack of sleep secondary to nighttime hot flashes. Emotional stress and the need to manage multiple responsibilities at work and home may result in an energy drain.

The quandary associated with FM is that people have paradoxical sleep patterns: they may sleep for extended periods of time without having refreshing sleep (Schaefer, 1995b). They believe their sleep patterns are normal but are told that they have a sleep disorder; it is the quality of sleep "that matters," not the length of time one sleeps.

Some research has indicated that disordered sleep patterns mark the origin of FM, but there are no magic potions to ensure consistent refreshed sleep for these women. Sleep may be improved by taking a warm bath or drinking warm milk before bedtime, by avoiding heavy foods for three to four hours before retiring, and by falling asleep to soothing music. A routine that is practiced on a daily basis is critical to the benefit of these interventions. One woman said, "If I go to bed too late or take my medicine later than normal, I end up feeling like I didn't sleep well and I begin to have some discomfort in my muscles." Women select those interventions that they believe they can perform while still maintaining some sense of control. If they feel out of control, the success of these interventions is undermined.

Although the notion of "routine" is important to these women, they need to recognize they may require additional sleep. During times of stress (e.g., deadlines at work, illness, menstrual periods), they may plan to get extra sleep at night or find a time when they can nap in the afternoon. If sleep is not possible, rest and relaxation, encouraged by slow rhythmic breathing and imagery, have the potential to replenish energy needs.

Additional concerns are self-care techniques such as vitamin therapy and special diets that the women believe may be the answer to their discomfort. They will often test whether certain foods, such as tomatoes or spices, will precipitate their symptoms. More drastic measures involve diets that are insufficient in the essential food groups. Severe weight loss, with potentially dangerous complications, can result. Women who lack accurate information about the disease itself may need referrals to nutritionists. The women should be encouraged to seek health care supervision if they choose to try a special diet.

Structural Integrity.   The maintenance of structural integrity is interwoven with the healing processes. Basic to structural integrity are a properly functioning immune system and an efficient inflammatory process for *fighting off* disease. Some women may have an elevated sedimentation rate, but many are frustrated because the diagnostic studies reveal no abnormality. There are a variety of responses to this process; each woman needs to know that, because of the uncertainty about the symptoms, other illnesses must be "ruled out" to ensure that appropriate interventions are ordered. This screening may place these patients at the mercy of the medical domination historically experienced by women (Ehrenreich & English, 1992).

Recognizing that the fears and uncertainty about why these tests are being performed constitute a normal response, nurses provide information and support. Nurses understand that a woman who just got married and is going through the diagnostic process may be worried about the range of possible problems and their effect on her marriage and perhaps her ability to have children. These fears are real and must be addressed. Helping the woman to live in the present may reduce her anticipatory fears. There is always a possibility that a cause may be identified and at least controlled now, and that a cure may be found in the near future.

Even without the support of causation, these women are frequently offered a variety of medications to help alleviate the symptoms associated with the disease. Clinical studies do not support a single approach, but a variety of drugs do produce some relief. When they do not, some women will seek help from homeopathy or herbal therapy—on their own, or with assistance from a trained clinician. Nursing implications include an assessment of the person's knowledge of the drug therapy and whether she is under expert care.

Patients taking antidepressants need to know about the possibility of weight gain, dry membranes, and constipation. Eating complex carbohydrates can help reduce the hunger associated with the increased serotonin levels. Drinking more water and eating a balanced diet may help reduce the dryness and constipation. Heart rate changes are associated with some of the antidepressants and should be reported to the physician or nurse practitioner. Patients sometimes sacrifice comfort because of fear associated with the side effects. They need reassurance that alternative medications are available if they cannot tolerate the prescribed drug. They need to be told that it might take some time to find a regimen that is most helpful, and that herbs and other over-the-counter remedies can be harmful and should not be taken without supervision.

To supplement the medication therapies, nurses can offer a variety of nontraditional approaches. Levine (1973b) encourages nurses to be creative in the maintenance of wholeness. Women, in particular, respond well to interventions such as relaxation, music, imagery, touch, presence, and massage.

Personal Integrity.   Concern for or maintenance of personal integrity reaffirms the importance of selfhood and self-esteem to an individual's oneness. Even though these women are making their voices heard, they frequently find themselves in an uncertain cycle that takes away whatever control they once had over their lives. Too often, their story rings true to the notion of "I was an active, vibrant, independent woman, and then, one day, all of that was gone. I lost my former self." Or, even worse, "I was no longer the person my husband married, so he left because he could not handle the changes." One woman expressed her devastation about her depression, her inability to work, and, in some occasions, her inability to go out of the house. Another woman recently indicated that she misses "my old self."

Nurses providing these women with options for self-care and insight to their difficulties will help them regain some of the control they believe they have lost. The women may need assistance dealing with their changed reality. Selder (1989) states that an individual who is unable to accept the changes and continues to try to recover the old reality will have more difficulty dealing with chronic illness than will a woman who has learned to live with the new reality. According to Levine (1991), health is not only the healing of an injured part but also the return to selfhood where the individual is free to pursue self-interests. Individuals who are helped and are willing to accept change can live productive lives with disabilities. How this help is achieved will depend on understanding the complexity of the individual who has the disability.

For some women, regaining a sense of selfhood means simply substituting something else for what was lost. One woman had to stop aerobic exercise because it began to make her feel worse rather than better. Exercise has been part of her lifestyle for over 20 years. Substituting a less stressful exercise such as walking gave her the possibility of continuing her daily exercise routine. Women need to understand that realization of the desired effects of any change or new intervention may take time. Having choices offers the option of selecting what they want to incorporate into their lifestyle, and this process of choice moves the women closer to their sense of selfhood and oneness. The women have fatigue and muscle pain, but they can find new ways to live with these changes. This process can be challenging and uplifting, provided there is support along the way. The women live with chronic uncertainty, which offers them the chance to see the challenges as opportunity and possibility (Mischel, 1990).

Social Integrity. The maintenance of social integrity acknowledges the person as a social being and recognizes the need to provide adequate attention to the family. Social support strengthens a woman's sense of self. All people have a basic need to be loved. When her husband leaves because the wife's illness is too much to bear, or friends drift away because the woman feels too miserable to be part of the group's activities, the woman wonders whether she will ever have a social life again.

The nurse can help these women find ways to maintain a social calendar that is not too tiring or stressful. Women tell a variety of stories: "I still take hikes. I just use a cane for support and take a little longer than normal. I don't mind being last in the pack." "My husband can't understand why I don't want to go camping anymore. He doesn't understand that I can't go all day like I used to. He wants to hike, go boating, and play games with the kids all in the same day." Some husbands/friends are understanding, some are not.

It is important to encourage the women to communicate openly and honestly. No one wants to hear a friend constantly complaining about his or her health, but these women need to let people know why they cannot do things as they did before. One woman talked about how her husband told her one day that he was sick and tired of hearing her talk about her illness all the time. She was shocked— and concerned that perhaps her problems were adversely affecting their marriage. She approached him to say that she was sorry but that sometimes she just needs to say that she's not feeling well. *Saying* that she does not feel well frees her to go on with whatever she can manage to do that day. He was feeling pressured to help her; she told him she did not expect him to help her to feel better; listening to her was enough. If open communication is difficult to achieve, referral to a counselor who can help the couple find renewed sharing can be beneficial.

Referral to support groups may be helpful for some women. A choice to continue with support group intervention is entirely up to each participant. It is helpful to ask, "How do I feel while I am there?" and "How do I feel after the meeting?" If the responses are positive, it may be advisable to continue with the support group. If the responses are negative, support group intervention may not be appropriate to that individual. For example, if a woman feels physically or emotionally worse after the meeting, it may be better to find support in other ways.

Alternatives to support groups include finding a friend or *buddy* who has the same problem and is willing to share mutual experiences. Women will often meet these friends at the support group meetings and casually develop a relationship with one person rather than with the group. For women who cannot attend support groups because of health or distance, on-line computer support or bulletin boards may be helpful. Supporting a woman's choices helps to improve her sense of self and maintain her wholeness.

Organismic Responses

The success of the interventions is measured through the observation of organismic responses. Although these interventions have not been tested empirically, responses observed in these women include: (a) reduction in reported pain or need for pain control, (b) reported improved quality of sleep, (c) reported improved ability to anticipate and plan for exacerbations, (d) better understanding of illness, (e) comfort in sharing of stories, (f) reduction in felt stress, and (g) reported improved functional status following adjustments in lifestyle. Responses that might be considered inappropriate adaptation include depression, increased fatigue, inability to socialize, and lack of restful sleep. Organismic responses that can be grounded in the experience of living with the illness include mastery of stress (personal integrity), function status (energy and structural integrity), quality of life (energy, structural, personal, and social integrity), and emotional well-being (all the integrities).

STRATEGIC PLANNING

When considering the implementation of a model for practice, it is important to address the following list of questions. Exploring the answers to these questions will assist nurses with determining the congruence between the Conservation Model and their beliefs about nursing, as well as the usefulness of the Conservation Model in their practice setting. These questions include the following:

1. On what assumptions is the model based? How consistent are these assumptions with my beliefs about nursing and nurses' role in health care? Do these assumptions hold true for the varieties of settings in which nurses function? Are they sufficiently robust to endure the changing nature of health care?

2. Is the language of the model universal and therefore usable by nurses from different cultural backgrounds? Is the language consistent with the language used by individuals who seek health care in the practice setting for which this model is being considered?

Except for the term trophicognosis, the language of the Conservation Model is easy to understand and use as a means of communication in a health care setting. Although conservation is a universal principle of life, a consultation with nurses from Norway revealed that there was no direct Norwegian equivalent for the word conservation (personal communication, June 3, 1991). Norwegian nurses attempting to use the model thought the word conservation meant conservative; to the contrary, the nurse uses creativity to improve care of the patient.

The term organismic responses might be confusing to some practicing nurses. The confusion increases when the responses are defined only as fight/flight, stress, immune, and perceptual responses. It is important to keep in mind that the organismic responses are not mutually exclusive and must be considered together as an integrated response. How these organismic responses are actually measured needs additional work. Both qualitative and quantitative studies will help to define more specifically the nature of the responses relative to avant-garde outcomes such as functional status and quality of life.

3. Are the goals of nursing consistent with the expectations of the patient? Is the patient concerned about maintaining integrity/wholeness? Empirical data support the concept that all human beings are concerned about their integrity even though they may not actively consider its significance until it is challenged beyond their ability to adapt.

4. Are the values inherent in the model consistent with the values held by the patient with chronic illness? Does the patient want to take part in the decisions about his or her health care? Does the patient want responsibility for selecting the most appropriate interventions? Is it important to have options from which to select? Consideration of cultural and social influences is extremely important to the delivery of care that meets the unique needs of individual patients.

5. Do nurses value human interaction? Do nurses perceive their role as one in which they provide care that is either therapeutic or supportive for the patient? Is the model flexible enough to promote creative interventions by nurses?

6. Do nurses place a value on the importance of research to the delivery of quality patient care? Is research part of practice or simply a mandate that must be reckoned with?

7. Is the model simple enough to be used by practicing nurses, yet parsimonious in its use with a variety of patients in a variety of settings?

8. Does the model provide direction for care of the patient in a community setting? Does the model tell nurses how to evaluate the effectiveness of the interventions?

TIPS FOR SUCCESS

Successful use of the Conservation Model is facilitated by learning how others have succeeded in implementating the model in their own practice or as a basis for nursing practice in an organization or on a patient care unit. Geist (personal communication, February 27, 1995) noted that lack of support from administrative personnel and incongruence with organizational goals make use of the model almost impossible. The following suggestions offer nurses additional tips for successful use of Levine's Conservation Model in practice.

1. Become familiar with the theorist and her work; read original works prior to reading others' interpretations of Levine's writings.
2. Determine your philosophy and beliefs about nursing, and match them with the assumptions and beliefs presented by the theorist.
3. Read papers in which the author(s) describe their use of the Conservation Model in education, research, administration, and clinical practice. Get a sense of how others have interpreted and used the model. Judge the appropriateness and accuracy of its use. Levine encourages others to continue to develop her model based on sound principles.
4. Read the research that has been completed using or testing the use of the model. Determine whether the findings have been appropriately integrated into the model. For example, Foreman's (1991) study of confusion in the elderly demonstrates the importance of considering all the conservation principles when the goal is to maintain wholeness. His work supports the use of the principles as a guide for determining interventions that will preserve wholeness.
5. Communicate with those who have used the model in their practice. Ask what problems they might have had and how

they dealt with them. Consider the problems you might encounter and how you would overcome them. Nurses who use
the framework are often very willing to be consulted.

6. Develop a detailed implementation plan with a strong emphasis on how the use of the model will improve patient care.

EVALUATING THE USE OF THE MODEL

If one assumes that the use of a nursing model to guide nursing will
help define the unique role of nursing in the health care arena, then
the outcomes of using the model should reflect the nurses' significant contributions. Consistent with Levine's Conservation Model,
the outcomes or significant contributions would be the maintenance of wholeness and the promotion of adaptation. However,
Levine (1991) has said that ". . . precise identification of the adaptive condition is not possible . . . the focus of nursing intervention
must be on the consequences of care rather than on algorithms designed to display the adaptive patterns. All discussions of adaptation
rest finally on generalizations arising from shared experience and
observations. The research necessary to describe adaptation patterns and the therapeutic interventions that will support them has
yet to be done" (pp. 6-7).

In her practice, the author keeps detailed records of observed and
reported responses to interventions. This is done with the patients'
full knowledge of her role as a researcher. These responses provide
insight to the adaptive responses shared by all the women.

IMPLEMENTATION

Direct care nurses, educators, and researchers continue to use the
Conservation Model as a way of organizing their practice and as a
basis for research. The model has been successfully used as the
basis of cardiovascular practice by Molchany (personal communication, January 12, 1995). This clinical nurse specialist states she uses
it often to address the diverse needs of cardiac patients, such as
individuals with myocardial rupture/ventricular septal defect
(Molchany, 1993), as well as the complex needs of families in crises

in the acute coronary setting. She has also found it to be very helpful in cardiovascular team rounds, as a way of organizing the discussion of interdisciplinary care. Ratachack (personal communication, January 26, 1995) finds it most helpful in ensuring the wholistic care of a patient admitted to a cardiac intensive care unit.

Stafford (personal communication, February 20, 1995) continues to use the model extensively in her cardiovascular practice to develop standards of care, identify nursing diagnoses, develop lectures for nursing students, and as the philosophical basis for discussing ethics in nursing practice. Winslow (personal communication, January 24, 1995) used the model as the basis of her dissertation, "Oxygen Consumption and Cardiovascular Response in Normal Subjects and in Acute Myocardial Infarction Patients During Basin Bath, Tub Bath, and Shower." Lane and Winslow (1987) expanded on these data in a later publication. Henrick (personal communication, February 21, 1995) used the Conservation Model to propose the development of a nurse-run clinic for men with congestive heart failure (CHF) who are at risk for readmission. Given the current focus on managed care, this proposal may have broad implications for care of both men and women with CHF living in the community. Early intervention can reduce cost of care by decreasing the frequency of required hospitalization.

Taylor (personal communication, February 22, 1995), although retired, used the conservation principles in managing the care of acutely ill patients with neurological challenges. She developed an assessment tool and nursing diagnoses for this group of complex patients, using the conservation principles as a guide (Taylor, 1989).

Foreman (1991) has used the Conservation Model as a structure to comprehensively examine the causes of and interventions (prevention and treatment) for acute confusion in elderly hospitalized patients. Cox (1991; personal communication, February 21, 1995) is using the conservation principles as a basis for her practice at the Alverno Health Care Facility. She is currently developing a program that focuses on the conservation of energy and structural integrity for Alzheimer's residents, and will soon be focusing on urinary incontinence. Happ (personal communication, January 31, 1995) is considering the use of the model in the care of the frail elderly in an acute care setting.

Pond (personal communication, January 29, 1995) continues to use the model as a basis for her own nurse-practitioner practice. She has found it to be useful and pragmatic in the care of women during pregnancy, as the basis of collaborative practice in the emergency room, in the care of the homeless, as a model for community health, and in the establishment of a primary care center for an underserved community. She notes, on many occasions, how much of nursing's work is grounded in the principles inherent in the model. Fleming (personal communication, February 23, 1995) continues to use the Conservation Model in her nurse midwifery practice. She believes that all midwives are using skills, techniques, and judgments—whether they know it or not—based on the conservation principles. She has demonstrated how the integration of the principles maintains the integrity of the women experiencing birthing.

The author has found that the language of the model is familiar to women in the community. Interventions to change a predicament or to provide comfort are consistent with their goals. She has successfully used the model as the basis of research that has examined fatigue in congestive heart failure (Schaefer, 1990; Schaefer & Potylycki, 1993) and sleep disturbance following coronary artery bypass surgery (Swavely, Schaefer, Rothenberger, Hess, & Williston, 1995).

The faculty at Allentown College of St. Francis de Sales use the model as a basis for the undergraduate and graduate programs. The model is sufficiently broad to incorporate changes that reflect a dynamic health care environment. For example, the model has provided the basis for health promotion, health maintenance, and supportive care in the community for sophomore and senior students.

Critique of the Conservation Model's use in community health is related to the lack of attention to epidemiology. Careful attention to the roots of the model will reveal that Nightingale's concern for sanitation is one of the fundamentals of the person–environment interaction. The principles of epidemiology as an adjunctive science provide important information about the risks, incidence, and prevalence of disease, and about the behaviors associated with industrial risk that are important sources of knowledge for the nurse providing care in the community. The information required is critical to understanding the environmental challenges to a community of individuals. One need only recall the environmental effects of Chernoble to understand how epidemiology impacts the provision of health care.

Names of nurse scholars who can provide assistance with curricular development are listed at the end of the chapter text.

CONCLUSION

Levine (1973a) developed her model with the intent of using it as a basis for organizing medical-surgical nursing in a way that would improve student learning. The model has a unique focus: the maintenance of wholeness and the promotion of adaptation in health and illness. The maintenance of wholeness is predicated on conservation, adaptation, and change. Nurses accomplish the goals inherent in the model by using the conservation principles (energy, structure, personal, and social integrity) to guide the development of plans of care. They work collaboratively with other health care providers to ensure that all aspects of patients' care are addressed, and they have a moral responsibility to encourage the patients' participation in their plans of care. The effect of care delivered is evaluated by observing for organismic responses. The model has been used successfully as the basis for research, and its usefulness in a variety of clinical practice settings with representative patient groups of all ages has been demonstrated.

CURRICULUM DEVELOPMENT:
NURSE SCHOLARS WHO CAN ASSIST

Ruth A. Cox, PhD, RN, OSF (long-term care; elderly)
President and CEO
The Alverno Health Care Facility
849 13th Avenue North
Clinton, IA 52732-5115
(319) 242-1521 (w)
(319) 242-7273 (h)
FAX (319) 243-3016

Nancy Fleming, PhD, CNM, RN (midwifery practice)
424 N. Adams
Hinsdale, IL 60524

Marquis D. Foreman, PhD, RN (confusion in the elderly; acute care)
Department of Medical-Surgical Nursing
College of Nursing (M/C 802)
University of Illinois at Chicago
845 South Damen Avenue
Chicago, IL 60612
(312) 966-8443 (w)
FAX (312) 996-4979

Deborah A. Geise, MS, CNM, RN (midwifery practice)
2801 6th Street
Monroe, WI 53566
(608) 325-4675 (h)
(608) 324-2146 (w)

Ann Henrick, PhD, RN, FAAN (public policy implications)
15 King Arthur #20
Northlake, IL 60164
(708) 343-7299, ext. 4305 (w)
(708) 562-8457 (h)
FAX (708) 216-2576

Constance Molchany, MSN, RN (cardiovascular nursing)
Cardiovascular Clinical Specialist
Lehigh Valley Hospital
Cedar Crest & I-78
Allentown, PA 18105
(610) 402-1714
(610) 402-8999 (page)

Jane Pond, CRNP, MSN, RNC (primary care; homeless; collaborative
    practice)
Assistant Professor/Director of Ambulatory Care Services
Temple University
3307 North Broad Street
Philadelphia, PA 19140
(215) 707-7879
E-mail JANEBP@ASTRO.OCIS.TEMPLE EDU

Sherry Ratajczak, MSN, RN (education; cardiovascular nursing)
Assistant Professor
Allentown College of St. Francis de Sales
2755 Station Avenue
Center Valley, PA 18034
(610) 282-1100, ext. 1397

Karen Moore Schaefer, DNSc, RN (cardiovascular nursing; education; chronic illness)
Associate Professor
Allentown College of St. Francis de Sales
2755 Station Avenue
Center Valley, PA 18034
(610) 282-1100, ext. 1285
E-mail SCHAEFER@ACCNOV.ALLENCOL.EDU

Margaret J. Stafford, MSN, RN, FAAN (cardiovascular nursing; nursing diagnosis)
21 King Arthur #1
Northlake, IL 60164
(708) 562-1378

Joyce Waterman Taylor, MSN, RN (neurological nursing; nursing diagnosis)
8265 Alston Avenue
Hesperia, CA 92345
(619) 948-2293 (h)

Elizabeth H. Winslow, PhD, RN, FAAN (cardiovascular nursing; critical care)
The University of Texas at Arlington
School of Nursing
P.O. Box 19407
Arlington, TX 76019
(817) 273-2776
FAX (817) 794-5006

ACKNOWLEDGMENTS

The author is grateful to Myra Levine for "publishing her ideas in the first place," and for her ongoing support and encouragement as she continued to work with the Conservation Model. She thanks Jane Benson Pond, MSN, CNP, RN, for her critical review of the manuscript, and Theresa Gyauch for her editorial contributions. She thanks all the nurse scholars who have shared their ideas and expertise in using the Conservation Model, and who have agreed to consult with other nurses about the use of the model.

REFERENCES

Bates, M. (1967). A naturalist at large. *Natural History, 76*(6), 8-16.

Beland, I. (1971). *Clinical nursing: Pathophysiological and psychosocial implications* (2nd ed.). New York: Macmillan.

Bennett, R. M., Clark, S. R., Goldberg, L., Nelson, D., Bonafede, R. P., Porter, J., & Specht, D. (1989). Aerobic fitness in patients with fibrositis. *Arthritis and Rheumatism, 32*(4), 454-460.

Bernard, C. (1957). *An introduction to the study of experimental medicine.* New York: Dover.

Boissevain, M. D., & McCain, G. A. (1991). Toward an integrated understanding of fibromyalgia syndrome: II. Psychological and phenomenological aspects. *Pain, 45,* 239-248.

Brunner, M. (1985). A conceptual approach to critical care nursing using Levine's model. *Focus on Critical Care, 12*(2), 39-44.

Cooper, D. H. (1990). Optimizing wound healing: A practice within nursing's domain. *Nursing Clinics of North America, 25*(1), 165-180.

Cox, R. A., Sr. (1991). A tradition of caring: Use of Levine's model in long-term care. In K. M. Schaefer & J. B. Pond (Eds.), *The conservation model: A framework for nursing practice* (pp. 179-197). Philadelphia: Davis.

Crawford-Gamble, P. E. (1986). An application of Levine's conceptual model. *Perioperative Nursing Quarterly, 2*(1), 64-70.

Daily, P. A., Bishop, G. D., Russell, I. J., & Fletcher, E. M. (1990). Psychological stress and the fibrositis/fibromyalgia syndrome. *Journal of Rheumatology, 17*(10), 1380-1385.

Dever, M. (1991). Care of children. In K. M. Schaefer & J. B. Pond (Eds.), *The conservation model: A framework for nursing practice* (pp. 71-82). Philadelphia: Davis.

Dibble, S. L., Bostrom-Ezrati, J., & Rizzuto, C. (1991). Clinical predictors of intravenous site symptoms. *Research in Nursing & Health, 14,* 413-420.

Dubos, R. (1965). *Man adapting.* New Haven, CT: Yale University Press.

Ehrenreich, B., & English, D. (1992). The "sick" women of the upper class. In C. Golden (Ed.), *The captive imagination: A casebook on the yellow wallpaper* (pp. 90–109). New York: Feminist Press.

Erickson, C. H. (1968). *Identity: Youth and crisis.* New York: Norton.

Fawcett, J. (1995). *Conceptual models of nursing* (3rd ed.). Philadelphia: Davis.

Foreman, M. D. (1991). Conserving cognitive integrity of the hospitalized elderly. In K. M. Schaefer & J. B. Pond (Eds.), *The conservation model: A framework for nursing practice* (pp. 133–150). Philadelphia: Davis.

Gibson, J. E. (1966). *The senses considered as perceptual systems.* Boston: Houghton Mifflin.

Goldstein, K. (1963). *The organism.* Boston: Beacon Press.

Grindley, J., & Paradowski, M. B. (1991). Developing an undergraduate program using Levine's model. In K. M. Schaefer & J. B. Pond (Eds.), *Levine's conservation model: A framework for nursing practice.* Philadelphia: Davis.

Hall, E. (1966). *The hidden dimension.* Garden City, NY: Doubleday.

Hirschfeld, M. H. (1976). The cognitively impaired older adult. *American Journal of Nursing, 76,* 1981–1984.

Inlander, C. (1992, April). Medical world strives to keep women "barefoot and dumb." *The Morning Call.*

Lane, L. D., & Winslow, E. H. (1987). Oxygen consumption, cardiovascular response, and perceived exertion in healthy adults during rest, occupied bedmaking, and unoccupied bedmaking activity. *Cardiovascular Nursing, 23*(6), 31–36.

Langer, V. S. (1990). Minimal handling protocol for the intensive care nursery. *Neonatal Network, 9*(3), 23–27.

Lentz, M. J., Shaver, J., & Heitkemper, M. (1993, November). Sleep alterations associated with somatic symptoms in midlife women. In J. Shaver (Chair), *Women's symptoms and stress: Person and environment factors.* Symposium conducted at the meeting of the American Nurses' Association Council of Nurse Researchers, Washington, DC.

Levine, M. E. (1966a). Adaptation and assessment: A rationale for nursing intervention. *American Journal of Nursing, 66,* 2450–2453.

Levine, M. E. (1966b). Trophicognosis: An alternative to nursing diagnosis. In *American Nurses' Association Regional Clinical Conference* (Vol. 2, pp. 55–70). New York: American Nurses Association.

Levine, M. E. (1968). Knock before entering personal space bubbles. *Chart,* 58–63.

Levine, M. E. (1969). The pursuit of wholeness. *American Journal of Nursing, 69,* 93–98.

Levine, M. E. (1971a). Holistic nursing. *Nursing Clinics of North America,* 6(2), 253-263.

Levine, M. E. (1971b). *Renewal for nursing.* Philadelphia: Davis.

Levine, M. E. (1973a). *Introduction to clinical nursing* (2nd ed.). Philadelphia: Davis.

Levine, M. E. (1973b). On creativity in nursing. *Image: The Journal of Nursing Scholarship, 3*(3), 15-19.

Levine, M. E. (1977). Nursing ethics and the ethical nurse. *American Journal of Nursing, 77*(5), 845-849.

Levine, M. E. (1984, August). Myra Levine. Paper presented at the Nurse Theorist Conference in Edmonton, Alberta. Canada. (cassette recording)

Levine, M. E. (1987). Approaches to the development of a nursing diagnosis taxonomy. In A. M. McLane (Ed.), *Classification of nursing diagnoses: Proceedings of the seventh conference* (pp. 45-60). St. Louis: Mosby.

Levine, M. E. (1988). Antecedents from adjunctive disciplines: Creation of nursing theory. *Nursing Science Quarterly, 1*(1), 16-21.

Levine, M. E. (1989a). Beyond dilemma. *Seminars in Oncology Nursing, 5,* 124-128.

Levine, M. E. (1989b). The ethics of nursing rhetoric. *Image: The Journal of Nursing Scholarship, 21*(1), 4-5.

Levine, M. E. (1989c). The conservation model: Twenty years later. In J. P. Riehl-Sisca (Ed.), *Conceptual models for nursing practice* (pp. 325-337). Norwalk, CT: Appleton & Lange.

Levine, M. E. (1989d). Ration or rescue: The elderly in critical care. *Critical Care Nursing, 12*(1), 82-89.

Levine, M. E. (1990). Conservation and integrity. In M. Parker (Ed.), *Nursing theories in practice* (pp. 189-201). New York: National League for Nursing.

Levine, M. E. (1991). The conservation model: A model for health. In K. M. Schaefer & J. B. Pond (Eds.), *The conservation model: A framework for nursing practice* (pp. 1-11). Philadelphia: Davis.

Levine, M. E. (1992). Nightingale redux. In F. Nightingale, *Notes on nursing: What it is, and what it is not* (Commemorative ed., pp. 39-43). Philadelphia: Lippincott.

Levine, M. E. (1994). Some further thoughts on nursing rhetoric. In J. F. Kiluchi & H. Simmons (Eds.), *Developing a philosophy of nursing* (pp. 104-109). Thousand Oaks, CA: Sage.

Littrell, K., & Schumann, L. (1989). Promoting sleep for the patient with a myocardial infarction. *Critical Care Nurse, 9*(3), 44-49.

Lynn-McHale, D. J., & Smith, A. (1991). Comprehensive assessment of families of the critically ill. In J. S. Leske (Ed.), *AACN Clinical Issues in Critical Care Nursing* (pp. 195–209). Philadelphia: Lippincott.

Martin, W. J. (1993). Two sides to every story. *Fibromyalgia Network, 21*, 8.

McCain, G. A., & Tilbe, K. S. (1989). Diurnal hormone variation in fibromyalgia syndrome: A comparison with rheumatoid arthritis. *Journal of Rheumatology, 19*, 154–157.

Mischel, M. H. (1990). Reconceptualization of the uncertainty in illness theory. *Image: The Journal of Nursing Scholarship, 22*(4), 256–262.

Molchany, C. A. (1993). Ventricular septal and free wall rupture complicating acute MI. *Journal of Cardiovascular Nursing, 6*(4), 38–45.

Moldofsky, H. (1989). Sleep-wake mechanisms in fibrositis. *Journal of Rheumatology, 84*, 47–48.

Newport, M. A. (1984). Conserving thermal energy and social integrity in the newborn. *Western Journal of Nursing Research, 6*(2), 175–197.

Nightingale, F. (1859). *Notes on nursing: What it is and what it is not.* London: Harrison & Sons.

O'Laughlin, K. M. (1986). Changes in bladder function in the woman undergoing radical hysterectomy for cervical cancer. *Journal of Obstetric, Gynecological, and Neonatal Nursing, 15*(5), 380–385.

Pasco, A., & Halupa, D. (1991). Chronic pain management. In K. M. Schaefer & J. B. Pond (Eds.), *The conservation model: A framework for practice* (pp. 101–117). Philadelphia: Davis.

Pond, J. B. (1991). Ambulatory care of the homeless. In K. M. Schaefer & J. B. Pond (Eds.), *The conservation model: A framework for practice* (pp. 167–178). Philadelphia: Davis.

Pond, J. B., & Taney, S. G. (1991). Emergency care in a large university emergency department. In K. M. Schaefer & J. B. Pond (Eds.), *The conservation model: A framework for practice* (pp. 151–166). Philadelphia: Davis.

Roberts, J. E., Fleming, N., & Yeates-Giese, D. (1991). Perineal integrity. In K. M. Schaefer & J. B. Pond (Eds.), *The conservation model: A framework for practice* (pp. 61–70). Philadelphia: Davis.

Rothchild, B. M. (1991). Fibromyalgia: An explanation for the aches and pains of the nineties. *Comprehensive Therapy, 17*(6), 9–14.

Savage, T. A., & Culbert, C. (1989). Early intervention: The unique role of nursing. *Journal of Pediatric Nursing, 4*(5), 339–345.

Schaefer, K. M. (1990). A description of fatigue associated with congestive heart failure: Use of Levine's Conservation Model. In M. E. Parker

(Ed.), *Nursing theories in practice* (pp. 217-237). New York: National League for Nursing.

Schaefer, K. M. (1991). Care of the patient with congestive heart failure. In K. M. Schaefer & J. B. Pond (Eds.), *The conservation model: A framework for practice* (pp. 119-132). Philadelphia: Davis.

Schaefer, K. M. (1995a). Struggling to maintain balance: A study of women with fibromyalgia. *Journal of Advanced Nursing, 21,* 95-102.

Schaefer, K. M. (1995b). Sleep and fatigue in women with fibromyalgia and chronic fatigue syndrome: A pilot study. *Journal of Obstetric, Gynecological, and Neonatal Nursing.*

Schaefer, K. M., & Potylycki, M. J. S. (1993). Fatigue associated with congestive heart failure: Use of Levine's Conservation Model. *Journal of Advanced Nursing, 18,* 260-268.

Selder, F. (1989). Life transition theory: The resolution of uncertainty. *Nursing & Health Care, 10*(8), 437-451.

Selye, H. (1956). *The stress of life.* New York: McGraw-Hill.

Shorter, E. (1992). *From paralysis to fatigue: A history of psychosomatic illness in the modern era.* New York: Free Press.

Swavely, D., Schaefer, K. M., Rothenberger, C., Hess, S., & Williston, D. (1995). *Sleep disturbances: Post-coronary artery surgery.* Manuscript submitted for publication.

Taylor, J. W. (1989). Levine's conservation principles. Using the model for nursing diagnosis in a neurological setting. In J. P. Riehl-Sisca (Ed.), *Conceptual models for nursing practice* (3rd ed., pp. 349-358). Norwalk, CT: Appleton & Lange.

Tribotti, S. (1990). Admission to the neonatal intensive care unit: Reducing the risks. *Neonatal Network, 8*(4), 17-22.

Waddington, C. H. (Ed.). (1968). *Towards a theoretical biology. I. Prolegomena.* Chicago: Aldine.

Webb, H. (1993). Holistic care following a palliative Hartmann's procedure. *British Journal of Nursing, 2*(2), 128-132.

Wolf, S. (1961). Disease as a way of life: Neural integration in systemic pathology. *Perspectives in Biology and Medicine, 4,* 288-305.

8

Application of Self-Care Deficit Nursing Theory

Ruben D. Fernandez, George J. Hebert, and Jane Bliss-Holtz

Implementation of a theory-based practice model for nursing entails the purposeful examination, identification, and articulation of values and beliefs relevant to care, patients, nursing, health, practice, management, and education. These values, as expressed by Newark Beth Israel's model and philosophy of practice, are consistent with the construct of the theory of Self-Care Deficit. Implementation of the theory has served to further expand the development of the conceptual framework. According to the Beth Israel experience, use of this theory has strengthened nursing practice, guided nursing care, and bridged the gap between nursing theory and nursing practice. [Written in support of all authors in Chapters 8 and 11.]

Dorothea E. Orem

The current health care environment offers unparalleled opportunities for hospitals and nursing services to redesign nursing care delivery toward high-quality, cost-effective care that will strengthen institutional alignment with the current and future customers.

The rapid rate of change, the turbulent environment, and the complexity of issues currently facing health care institutions and nursing systems have the potential to create reactive responses. Nursing services are experiencing a sense of urgency and pressure from external forces. Unfortunately, the demand to respond may result in developing short-term, less adequate approaches to restructuring work roles and relationships, and these approaches may undermine care values and principles of nursing care. As nursing transforms the future through redesign, managed competition, managed care, high quality, and cost efficiency, it is imperative that the response be coordinated, systematic, formalized, developed, and implemented based on careful consideration of professional, ethical, financial, and sociotechnical principles.

At Newark Beth Israel Medical Center, we rejected quick-fix solutions and embarked on a planned, calculated change project that encompassed work redesign and theory-based practice. We committed ourselves to implementing Dorothea E. Orem's Self-Care Deficit Nursing Theory as the framework for professional practice.

A theory-based practice model for nursing provides the structure for understanding all the practice components of nursing service delivery. The model lays the foundation for nursing practice by providing a framework that organizes knowledge, and delivery of care based on that knowledge, thus creating a bridge between nursing theory and nursing practice (Fernandez, Hebert, & Riggs, 1995; Fernandez & Wheeler, 1990).

Theory-based practice is a high-level motivator that provides structure and cohesion for nursing. Theory clarifies the nurse–patient relationship and the parameters for nursing practice. Deriving practice from a conceptually developed theory of nursing maximizes the possibility of conceptual consistency in practice and the potential for bringing order to nurses' experience and knowledge (Taylor, 1988).

The need for practice-oriented theory and conceptual models for nursing practice has been identified in the nursing literature for many years. However, the implementation of a conceptual model has been difficult because of the values of the health care industry, the incongruence of hospital systems, medical models superimposed on nursing practice, lack of understanding of the phenomenon of nursing, and the absence of a clearly articulated practice-oriented theory.

The Self-Care Deficit Nursing Theory originated from Orem's observation of nurses during her tenure as a nursing consultant for the Division of Hospital and Institutional Services of the Indiana State Board of Health from 1949 to 1957. Work continued over the years through the Nursing Model Committee of the Catholic University Nursing Faculty in 1965, and the Nursing Development Conference Group in 1968 (Fawcett, 1989; Nursing Development Conference Group, 1973; Orem & Taylor, 1986).

Self-Care Deficit Nursing Theory answers the questions of when nursing is needed and by whom, and what nursing practice procedures are necessary. Thus, it is a practice model. Within the model, Orem (1991) defines the operations of nursing practice very clearly. This model was congruent with the needs specified during the search for an appropriate model on which to base nursing practice at Newark Beth Israel Medical Center. In a document written in 1990 as a proposal for the New Jersey Department of Health Nursing Incentive Reimbursement Program, Fernandez and Riggs stated that Self-Care Deficit Nursing Theory went beyond a simple description of nursing tasks to identify and match nursing care resources with individual patient needs within a rigorous, coherent framework (p. 93).

Orem's general theory integrates the theory of self-care, the theory of self-care deficit, and the theory of nursing systems, which also defines the focus of nursing.

The concepts of the theory are: Therapeutic Self-Care Demand, Self-Care Agency, Basic Conditioning Factors, Self-Care Deficit, and Nursing Systems. The subconcepts are Universal Self-Care Requisites, Developmental Self-Care Requisites, Health Deviation Self-Care Requisites, Foundational Capabilities and Dispositions, Power Components, and Self-Care Operations.

The basic proposition of the theory is that the Therapeutic Self-Care Demand is equal to the Self-Care Agency in persons who do not need nursing intervention. The Therapeutic Self-Care Demand is comprised of three requisites:

1. Universal Self-Care Requisites. These requisites are common to all humans across the life cycle.
2. Developmental Self-Care Requisites. These requisites include requisites related to promoting and maintaining development, to preventing developmental delays, and to mitigating or overcoming existing developmental delays.
3. Health Deviation Self-Care Requisites. These requisites are associated with dealing with health care system factors—factors generated through contact with the health care system. Health care system factors include such elements as medical diagnoses, treatments prescribed by other health care professionals, medication orders, and diagnostic tests.

Self-Care Agency is composed of Foundational Capabilities and Dispositions Power Components, and Self-Care Operations. Foundational Capabilities and Dispositions are the learned and innate capabilities needed specifically to perform actions related to maintaining health and development. There are three types of Self-Care Operations—estimative, transitional, and productive—and they are directly related to specific requisites and are the actions needed to fulfill particular requisites. Basic Conditioning Factors affect both the Therapeutic Self-Care Demand and the Self-Care Agency of an individual (Orem, 1991).

The structure of the model has been described above. As the institution was reviewing models that were articulated enough to define nursing practice and also were based on a philosophy of self-care, this model related well to the vision of nursing practice as held by the Department of Nursing.

Assumptions underlying the theory include (Orem, 1985, 1991):

1. Individuals value their ability to care for themselves and normally will do so without intervention from health care professionals;
2. People are responsible for themselves and will seek help when they cannot meet their requisites;
3. The health care system values people's perspective about their own health;

4. The roles of the person and the health care provider should be negotiated and acceptable to both parties.

Implementing a theoretical base in redesigning nursing care entails the identification, purposeful examination, and clear articulation of beliefs and values relevant to patients, nursing, health care, management, education, and nursing care. These values must be formulated into a specific philosophy of care that can be used to direct the development of a conceptual framework that will strengthen professional nursing practice and guide nursing care delivery within the institution.

Organizing a nursing department through theory-based practice responds to the current and future needs of patients and nurses. Furthermore, it responds to the need to operate in concert while focusing on a common purpose. Orem's Self-Care Deficit Nursing Theory best met the needs of the department because the theory:

1. Provides a common language.
2. Identifies a framework based on concepts unique to the discipline of nursing.
3. Provides a structure for decision making.
4. Directs nursing actions.
5. Allows nurses to practice nursing as a learned profession.
6. Provides a structure for the generation of new knowledge.
7. Reflects the values of the staff and the philosophy of the nursing department.
8. Can be utilized to justify nursing actions.
9. Provides a structure that the nursing department can use to operationalize its action plan.
10. Can cost out those interventions that are germane to nursing practice.
11. Provides a values system and practice identity that the staff can identify with, integrate, and interpret to others.
12. Can be utilized within a case management strategy to:
    a. Develop a resource utilization standard for each nursing diagnosis process.

   b. Compare the resources used for each individual patient with the resource utilization standard for care of the patient with a primary diagnosis.

   c. Analyze the variation from the standard to determine its cause.

   d. Facilitate performance of research within the process of case management.

Nursing administration agreed that, to make the project a success, certain investments were required (Fernandez & Wheeler, 1990): a dedicated specialist in Orem's nursing theory had to be hired as project facilitator; additional human resources had to be allocated for the purposes of education and implementation; an Orem resource library had to be developed; and the nursing department had to become known locally and nationally as an Orem center of nursing excellence and practice.

The designated investment goals were put into operation. An Orem coordinator was originally hired to spearhead the project; this position has now been replaced with an Orem consultant and facilitator. A blueprint was formulated with a target date of 5 years to establish and integrate the model. At this point, 6 years into the model, the department is in an active phase of implementation. Nursing administration is conscious that this process is ongoing, but, in order to evaluate goal attainment, time tables had to be established. Continuous quality-improvement programs and staff development programs were needed, to reflect the totality of the model. Policies and procedures, as they were revised and updated, incorporated the concepts and principles of the Self-Care Deficit Nursing Theory. In addition, the nursing department is committed to sponsor the Eastern Region Orem Self-Care Deficit Conferences, which are held biannually. To date, five regional conferences have been held, as well as research symposia.

The vision and the 5-year blueprint called for the development of an Orem-based computer system. The department elected to sponsor and provide access to Nursing System International in developing the first Orem theory-based computerized nursing system. The medical center became the first nursing department to contract services, provide data, and become a national testing and demonstration center for the purpose of advancing development of the model.

For a theory-based practice model to effectively operate, a multi-level forum must exist through which ongoing evaluation, free discussion, and planning can take place. The communication process must encompass the unit level, middle management, and the senior executive level. The overall concerns of the staff, the action plan, and the vision and mission must be clearly outlined and reiterated during each phase of the implementation process.

The implementation process (Fernandez, Hebert, & Riggs, 1995; Fernandez & Wheeler, 1990) includes but is not limited to five major phases:

Phase 1: Identification (2–8 months). This phase includes selection of a theory-based practice model.

Phase 2: Education (2–4 years). Although the process is ongoing, everyone in the department must be educated and have a good understanding of the model. This process includes the education department and other services external to nursing.

Phase 3: Transition (4–6 years). The staff has various levels of understanding and facility with the model. As they incorporate the theory into their daily activities, progress is made in documentation. Tools continue to be developed, expanded, and revised.

Phase 4: Implementation (6–8 years). The model is fully operational, and changes in practice and outcomes are evident. Tools of practice are near completion or completed. The staff practices according to the model, and true integration begins to occur.

Phase 5: Evaluation. Although the evaluation process is dynamic and ongoing, it is imperative that a thorough evaluation of the program be undertaken after completion of the implementation phase. Included is a review of compliance with preestablished goals, patient care outcomes, changes in practice, and movement toward theory integration. The theory is further refined by those staff members who understand it and have integrated it into their practice.

The implementation of theory-based practice at Newark Beth Israel Medical Center illustrates how a department can be organized and structured to face the demands of today's fluid health care system. Nursing leaders need to meet the challenge, chart a blueprint for action, and take the necessary risks to make things happen. Success belongs to those leaders and organizations that are capable of not only seeing the future but charting it.

REFERENCES

Fawcett, J. (1989). *Analysis and evaluation of conceptual models in nursing* (2nd ed.). Philadelphia: Davis.

Fernandez, R., Hebert, G., & Riggs, J. (1995). Transformational leadership: The partnership of theory-based practice and work redesign in a nursing care delivery model. In D. Flarey (Ed.), *Redesigning nursing care delivery: Transforming our future.* Philadelphia: Lippincott.

Fernandez, R., & Riggs, J. (1990). *Proposal for work redesign and the implementation of computer support of theory-based practice.* Trenton: New Jersey State Department of Health.

Fernandez, R., & Wheeler, J. (1990). Organizing a nursing system through theory-based practice. In G. Mayer, M. Madden, & E. Lawrenz (Eds.), *Patient care delivery models.* Rockville, MD: Aspen.

Nursing Development Conference Group. (1973). *Concept formalization in nursing. Process and product* (2nd ed.). Boston: Little, Brown.

Orem, D. E. (1985). *Nursing: Concepts of practice* (3rd ed.). New York: McGraw-Hill.

Orem, D. E. (1991). *Nursing: Concepts of practice* (4th ed.). St. Louis: Mosby.

Orem, D. E., & Taylor, S. (1986). Orem's general theory of nursing. In P. Winstead-Fry (Ed.), *Case studies in nursing theory* (pp. 37–71). New York: National League for Nursing.

Taylor, S. G. (1988). Nursing theory and nursing practice: Orem's theory in practice. *Nursing Science Quarterly, 1*(3), pp. 111–119.

9

The Riehl Interaction Model

Joan Riehl

*T*he Riehl Interaction Model has been implemented throughout the United States and in Canada, England, Europe, and Asia. The functional areas of choice have included all aspects of nursing: administration, education, practice, and research. This chapter describes its implementation in practice.

EXPLANATION OF THE MODEL

Philosophical Underpinnings

As the name of the model implies, its philosophy has social-psychological underpinnings and refers to any interaction occurring between two people, or one person and a group, or two or more groups. An assessment tool demonstrates how the physical, biological, social, and behavioral sciences are addressed. Throughout a given relationship, emphasis is placed on the *interaction* of all parts/parties involved, whether they are individuals or groups.

The model gives the practicing nurse guidelines for the best possible comprehensive care. Adherence to the guidelines is facilitated by understanding and implementing *symbolic interactionism,* which is the underlying philosophy of the Riehl Interaction Model.

Only a few key elements are presented here. Readers are referred to original sources—e.g., Riehl-Sisca (1989)—for more detail. Mead (1934) was an early proponent of symbolic interactionism. Rose (1962, 1980) identified the analytic and genetic assumptions of symbolic interactionism that form the basic assumptions in the Riehl Interaction Model. Blumer (1969) emphasized the importance of "getting inside" individuals' defining processes, in order to understand the symbols and meanings that comprise their world. He proposed five philosophical premises that complemented Rose's work and are utilized in the Riehl Interaction Model (Riehl-Sisca, 1989).

Analytic Assumptions. Rose's *Analytic Assumptions* illustrate how a nurse uses this information, and they explore the significance of symbols:

1. Symbolic as well as physical environments stimulate a nurse to act in caring for a patient; for example, a patient may not complain verbally of pain but grimaces whenever it is necessary to move in bed. Often, a person does not act but simply reacts; without thinking, the person responds. Response is especially evident when actions become habitual. In observing a patient's nonverbal communication, the nurse anticipates these reactions and makes the patient more comfortable by providing comprehensive care.

2. Through symbols, people stimulate other persons in ways that differ from those in which they themselves are stimulated.

3. Through symbols communicated by others, people can learn huge numbers of meanings, values, and ways of acting.

4. The meanings and values to which symbols refer do not occur in isolated bits but are present in large and complex clusters.

5. Thinking is the process by which symbolic solutions and actions are examined, assessed for their advantages and

disadvantages (in terms of the values of the individual). One "best" action is then chosen.

Genetic Assumptions.   Rose's Genetic Assumptions include:

1. The presence of a society, defined as a network of interacting individuals who share cultures, meanings, and values. The society takes precedence over any existing individual.
2. A process of internal socialization, which takes place in stages in the development of the infant.
3. A process of external socialization, which occurs in the general culture and within the various subcultures.
4. The survival, however subtle, of old groups, cultural expectations, and personal meaning and values; although they seem to have been dropped, they are not lost or forgotten.

The first Analytic Assumption is clearly relevant to nursing. The remaining assumptions, although more loosely related, are easily adaptable to nursing.

The element of human conduct relates to the meaning a given situation has for a particular individual. Role taking is then inferred. For example, the nurse must understand the meaning of a given situation for the client/patient by taking the role of that person. By attempting to see things from the client/patient's perspective, the nurse bases the eventual action on validated observations.

A sense of self, or a *self* concept, is another key element of the model. The use of self by the nurse in interpersonal interaction assists the client/patient in defining the situation. The client and nurse can then jointly interpret and clarify the meaning of an experience. Blumer (1969) has emphasized the importance of interpreting the actions of others rather than reacting to them.

These concepts and subconcepts are applicable in a thorough initial assessment of a client/patient. In the assessment process, the nurse incorporates knowledge from the physical, biological, social, and behavioral sciences. Knauth and Gross (1989) use the terminology of physiological, sociocultural, situational, environmental, and psychological disciplines in their assessment tool, which is based on the Riehl Interaction Model. As childbirth educators, Knauth and

Gross found the Riehl Interaction Model to be most helpful in their practice.

MODEL CONCEPTS AND PROCESSES

The concepts and subconcepts of the Riehl Interaction Model emerge directly from the philosophy discussed and briefly described above. Person, Environment, Nursing, and Health are inherent in the nurse—client/patient interaction. For example, the Person is genetically and socially an emerging, developing, changing self. The surrounding Environment influences and interacts with internal and external factors of the self. Nursing is the therapeutic process that guides the nurse–client/patient interaction toward its greatest health potential. Health is a wellness–illness process monitored by a person's view of self, which, in turn, is influenced by information received from self, others, and role relationships.

Affiliations among the model concepts, and their transferability into political and cultural environments or practice situations, can be readily transferred into a worldview. Political and cultural environments involve people interacting at various levels. For example, in national politics in the United States, the presidential candidates of the Democratic Party, the Republican Party, and any independent parties campaign against each other. Each Party acts as one entity, in much the same way an individual does in any given situation. When the campaign is over, the winner and his Party must negotiate compromises with members of the other parties if any progress is to be made.

The model's concepts are *all* interrelated in their emergence from symbolic interactionism in sociology. Because it has an identified sociocultural base, the model can be well utilized in various cultural settings where the uniqueness of self concepts and of the roles inherent in all individuals and societies are taken into account.

Similar to politics, cultural environments undergo changes; often, they are dramatically evident from one generation to the next. For example, the younger generation may be rebellious against the older, traditional ways of their parents and grandparents. Among young people, there is a great need to be accepted by peers, whose habits, dress, and preferences are often imitated and adopted over parental objection. Mass media content and advertising promulgate the desirability of these changes globally.

Redfield (1994), in *The Celestine Prophecy,* illustrates the importance of the self concept and the resultant roles that people take in any given situation. He identifies four personality types: (a) intimidator, (b) interrogator, (c) aloof, and (d) "poor me." Each type is labeled according to the roles taken by persons at some time in their life.

In all social interactions, self concepts and role assumptions become evident. Throughout this chapter, illustrations explain the application of symbolic interactionism in nursing practice.

The Riehl Interaction Model has been implemented in numerous clinical settings. Some examples include: the utilization of personal space by clients in a clinic environment (Foster, 1989), the self concept of a child with diabetes (Stumpf, 1989), the use of the model with a woman needing a mastectomy and a man with a myocardial infarction (Aggleton & Chalmers, 1989), and the practical application of the model, by staff and clients, in a mother-and-baby psychiatric unit (Arumugam, 1989).

The structure of the model, which allows its functional relationship to nursing practice, utilizes the physiological, sociocultural, situational, environmental and psychological aspects described above by Knauth and Gross. Practitioners utilizing the Riehl Interaction Model employ the mnemonic FANCAP, which represents *F*luids, *A*eration, *N*utrition, *C*ommunication, *A*ctivity, and *P*ain. These terms identify potential problems and give direction for ranking health problem areas with the patient and family.

A nursing staff's implementation of this model is well illustrated by Arumugam (1989), who first utilized the Riehl Interaction Model with families and staff of an inpatient unit of a psychiatric hospital in Manchester, England. The practitioner (Arumugam) employed the Riehl Interaction Model with both families and staff. A second utilization took place in two hospitals, in Bristol and in Bath, England (Aggleton & Chalmers, 1989). A third group of patients was seen at a university hospital in Hershey, Pennsylvania, where two childbirth educators (Knauth & Gross, 1989) applied the Riehl Interaction Model in caring for prenatal clients. Another practitioner and administrative department head in a Johnstown, Pennsylvania, clinic setting focused on nursing research and used the model in practice (Foster, 1989).

FITTING THE CONCEPTUAL MODEL TO THE PRACTICE SETTING

Use in nursing practice was the original purpose and function for which the Riehl Interaction Model was developed. In the front matter of each edition of her book, *Conceptual Models for Nursing Practice* (1989), Riehl states her underlying philosophy by quoting Kant: "Experience without theory is blind but theory without experience is mere intellectual play."

Because symbolic interaction is broad in scope and applicable beyond the profession of nursing, the Riehl conceptual approach can be used among a wide variety of clients. Aggleton and Chalmers (1989) illustrate usage in two different situations: one patient was admitted to the hospital for a mastectomy, and the other had a myocardial infarction.

The model's use in research is demonstrated by Stumpf (1989), who examined the self concept of children with diabetes (age range: 6 to 12 years). Stumpf focused on the relationship of the children's self concept to the control of their blood glucose. In this study, a group approach was necessary for a comprehensive analysis of the data.

Utilization of this model in education is illustrated by Riehl (Riehl-Sisca, 1989). She advocates that several class sessions be provided for students to best comprehend the concepts involved and their implementation into practice. Although the author suggests presenting the content in a prescribed depth and order, another instructor might choose a different approach, dictated by the learning level of the students. For beginning students, a somewhat simplified plan would be required. Small groups of students have demonstrated use of the model in a wide variety of community settings and clinical specialty areas.

Use of the Riehl Interaction Model in nursing administration has been demonstrated by Foster (1989). At the time of this writing, Foster is an administrative department head in a Family Medical

Center where patients' uses of personal space in a clinic setting have been observed.

COMPLEXITY OF THE RIEHL INTERACTION MODEL

Although the model has several related concepts and is somewhat broad in scope, it has proven valid for implementation in a variety of practice settings, as reflected in the literature. Model complexity should be rated seven on a scale from one (simple) to ten (complex). An understanding of the concepts of the model *must* precede its implementation into nursing practice. The concepts inherent in symbolic interactionism will apply in territorial situations and those requiring a worldview.

Accessibility of Riehl Interaction Model Experts

The author is the primary resource and welcomes contact from nurses. Those who have implemented the model under the guidance of the author could consult on its application to practice and advise on its use.

Time, Cost, and Training Factors

1. Successful education on the elements of the model is related to learning the underlying theory from trainers.
2. Group learning could be cost-effective, and the expense could be subsumed into the inservice education budget in a Nursing Service Department and/or included in the cost of the faculty in a School of Nursing.
3. Time would vary with the educational and interest level of the group being trained, and with the purpose of implementation. No actual financial figures have been factored out as yet.

Assessment of the Model in Use

The purpose of a comprehensive assessment is to identify any problems that may exist in addition to the primary concern of the client/patient. These secondary factors may be contributing to the problem at hand. Once all problems are identified, the nurse fulfills the remaining steps of the nursing process: making a plan of care, implementing it, evaluating it, and doing a reassessment as needed.

The assessment tool for the Riehl Interaction Model uses FANCAP—*F*luids, *A*eration, *N*utrition, *C*ommunication, *A*ctivity, and *P*ain—as a guide. FANCAP data may be obtained as follows: a physiological FANCAP; a sociocultural, situation, and environmental FANCAP; and a psychological FANCAP. Some vital statistics may also be obtained, as required in particular situations (Knauth & Gross, 1989).

Arumugam (1989) supplemented his assessment with such entries as Medical Status, Psychosocial Problems, Role and Role Flexibility, and Problem Solving. This approach helped him in working with psychiatric patients and the hospital staff. Perhaps these categories could have been as easily subsumed under the groupings used by Knauth and Gross. However, a philosophical premise inherent in the model is that human conduct is based on the meaning of the situation *for the person,* and role theory is a basic component (Riehl, 1989). Some latitude can therefore be employed by different practitioners in differing situations. As already mentioned, Aggleton and Chalmers (1989) used the model successfully in care plans for a married woman who needed a mastectomy and a 54-year old male patient with a diagnosis of myocardial infarction. The perceived problems were identified and discussed.

Foster's (1989) strategy engaged a research methodological approach in problem identification and patient care. In reviewing symbolic interactionism, which contains the philosophical underpinnings for the Riehl Interaction Model, Foster discusses the beliefs of Mead, Rose, and Blumer, who proposed these concepts, and she relates these data to spatial behavior within the domain of both the patient and the nurse. She emphasizes role relationships as a key component of the Riehl Interaction Model.

Assessing the Organizational Setting

The challenge of correct assessment is the choice of the nurse in practice. When Arumugam first used the Riehl Interaction Model in 1984 to deliver nursing care to patients in a rehabilitation unit, the model helped make nursing actions more meaningful (Arumugam,

1989). He stated that "it shifted my personal perspective from a be-havioral to a symbolic interactionism approach. I began to appreci-ate the model's potential usefulness in an acute psychiatric environment" (p. 413).

Language and Assumptions of the Model

A practicing nurse who wishes to understand the language and underlying philosophy of the model is encouraged to read the origi-nal sources from which it was derived: Mead (1934), Rose (1962, 1980), and Blumer (1969). Many potential questions will thereby be resolved. This research may be particularly important for nurses in other countries.

Planning for Implementation

Nursing models have been in use for more than twenty years. Among the considerations that have enhanced this use is the fact that the models were taught in nursing schools and were gradually utilized in nursing practice. As utilization increased, nurses began to include them as part of their patient care. Advanced nursing edu-cation, and support by colleagues and nursing leaders, helped facili-tate model use. A few models existed when the Riehl Interaction Model was developed. Nurses incorporated the Riehl Interaction Model into their nursing care on the basis of philosophic similarities and utility of concepts.

Resources have been available to answer questions. However, when the model was first developed, the author anticipated many potential questions and resolved them during the model's imple-mentation into practice. As questions arose, answers were consoli-dated to give the model further refinement.

Readers who are reporting on or trying to implement the Riehl In-teraction Model should *first* read the examples given in *Conceptual Models for Nursing Practice* (Riehl-Sisca, 1989). If further clarifica-tion is necessary, the author and other users of the Riehl Interaction Model welcome contact from nurses. As implementations increase in practice settings, the model will continue to be refined. To date, the model has consistently fulfilled its original purpose of use in practice.

Congruency of the model with goals in nursing practice is reflected in the functional areas discussed earlier in this chapter.

Analysis of Tasks Performed and People Implementing the Model

1. The initial task needed to implement the model was the completion of an assessment of the patients or populations involved. This was accomplished by a nurse in practice. An assessment tool was derived from this experience.

2. The educational level of the target audience (the patient) mattered not, as long as the questions being asked by the practitioner were understood. If the client did not understand the language used by the nurse, an interpreter would intercede in order to ensure that accurate messages were conveyed between the patient and nurse in the practice situation. This process was repeated throughout the implementation of the care plan, to guarantee that the plan was followed.

3. Support for practitioners has been available from the author since inception of the model. Clarification of any aspects of the model and its use has been effected through the media and personal communication.

4. The objectives to be achieved in implementation of the Riehl Interaction Model in practice were: to provide for practicing nurses an organized structure that would assist and guide them in giving the best possible comprehensive care to their clients; to contribute to the science of nursing; and to provide a nursing practice model that would complement, in approach, other models in use for client care.

5. An implementation time line is usually established for staff education, development of specific tools, and follow-up support and resources.

The author developed and selected the tools for this model, and they were available for use by practitioners since the outset. The learning time for the nurses varied, depending on the resources available and the purpose for the model's use. Familiarity with the implementation tools and approach is a by-product of learning to use the Riehl Interaction Model. Skill in using the tools increases with use. Tasks were assigned as appropriate, when the model was implemented in an organizational setting.

As with all nursing care assignments, tasks are goals directed toward meeting the needs of the patients. These include executing the doctors' orders and following the expectations on the ward in a hospital setting. Some latitude is provided in caring for patients, which permits the nurse to implement the nursing model chosen. Giving periodic reports provides an opportunity to educate other nurses about the model—and the approach needed in caring for patients. Descriptions of increasing success will stimulate the interest of other nurses and initiate a desire to utilize the model and gain similar benefits. In clinical situations, it is important to gain approval (or sanction) of the plan of care from the supervisor of the Nursing Service Department.

Ensuring Successful Model Implementation

The following tips are directed toward readers who are interested in implementing the Riehl Interaction Model. The most important advice is: Be thoroughly familiar with the model and how it is to be utilized *before* initiating its use. Be certain that the person(s) using it really like and believe in the model and can visualize its capacity to deliver the best possible care to patients.

After nurses have learned this model, including its theoretical philosophy and implementation tools, and have chosen it as a guide to providing improved nursing practice, no integrity-type problems have surfaced. The primary reason for this, I believe, is that practitioners who have chosen this particular model sincerely want and accept guidance in giving care as professional nurses. Questions that have arisen have been discussed and resolved with resource personnel.

Evaluation of the Model in Practice

Evaluation is accomplished by using formative and summative processes. Both types of processes have been applied in the Riehl Interaction Model. A demonstration is given by Aggleton and

Chalmers (1989), who used the model in practice and validated the functional area discussed here. Formative and summative evaluations are broad enough to be generalized to other functional areas.

Knauth and Gross (1989) also offered an evaluation of their care as childbirth educators in a clinical setting and a step-by-step follow-up of the interventions they implemented. The Riehl Interaction Model fits well the profile of caring that has historically been an important aspect of nursing.

REFERENCES

Aggleton, P., & Chalmers, H. (1989). Working with the Riehl model of nursing. In J. Riehl-Sisca (Ed.), *Conceptual models for nursing practice* (3rd ed.). Norwalk, CT: Appleton & Lange.

Arumugam, U. (1989). The Riehl model in practice: With families and with staff. In J. Riehl-Sisca (Ed.), *Conceptual models for nursing practice* (3rd ed.). Norwalk, CT: Appleton & Lange.

Blumer, H. (1969). *Interactionism: Perspective and method.* Englewood Cliffs, NJ: Prentice-Hall.

Foster, R. M. (1989). The nursing role, symbolic interactionism, and the patient's personal space. In J. Riehl-Sisca (Ed.), *Conceptual models for nursing practice* (3rd ed.). Norwalk, CT: Appleton & Lange.

Knauth, D. G., & Gross, E. B. (1989). The Riehl Interaction Model prenatal family assessment tool for the childbirth educator. In J. Riehl-Sisca (Ed.), *Conceptual models for nursing practice* (3rd ed.). Norwalk, CT: Appleton & Lange.

Mead, G. H. (1934). *Mind, self and society.* Chicago: University of Chicago Press.

Redfield, J. (1994). *The celestine prophecy.* New York: Warner Books.

*Riehl-Sisca, J. (Ed.). (1989). *Conceptual models for nursing practice* (3rd ed.). Norwalk, CT: Appleton & Lange.

Riehl-Sisca, J. (1989). The Riehl Interaction Model: An update. In J. Riehl-Sisca (Ed.), *Conceptual models for nursing practice* (3rd ed.). Norwalk, CT: Appleton & Lange.

* *Editor's Note: Conceptual Models for Nursing Practice* (2nd ed.) was translated into Japanese. *Conceptual Models for Nursing Practice* (3rd ed.) was translated into Spanish.

Rose, A. M. (1962). *Human behavior and social processes.* Boston: Houghton Mifflin.

Rose, A. M. (1980). A systematic summary of symbolic interaction theory. In J. P. Riehl & C. Roy (Eds.), *Conceptual models for nursing practice* (2nd ed.). New York: Appleton-Century-Crofts.

Stumpf, L. R. (1989). Self-concept of the child with diabetes: Its relationship to control of blood glucose. In J. Riehl-Sisca (Ed.), *Conceptual models for nursing practice* (3rd ed.). Norwalk, CT: Appleton & Lange.

RESOURCE CONTACTS

Peter Aggleton, PhD, MEd, MA, ABPSS
Senior Lecturer in Education
Bristol Polytechnic
Bristol, England

School of Nursing
Neumann College
Aston, Pennsylvania

Utharas Arumugam, DipN, RMN
School of Nursing
North Manchester General
   Hospital
Crumpsall, Manchester, England

Donna G. Knauth, MS, RN
Perinatal Clinical Nurse
   Specialist and Clinical
   Coordinator in Maternity
Riverview Medical Center
Red Bank, New Jersey

Helen Chalmers, SRN, DipN,
   RNT, BA
Senior Nurse Tutor
Bath District Health Authority
Bath, England

Joan Riehl, PhD, MA, MS, RN
Author, Lecturer, Consultant
P. O. Box 34405
Los Angeles, California

Rose Marie Foster, MSN, RN
Administrative Department
   Head
Family Medical Center
Conamough Valley Memorial
   Hospital
Johnstown, Pennsylvania

Linda R. Stumpf, MSN, RN
Case Manager
Forbes Health System
Monroeville, Pennsylvania

Ella B. Gross, MSN, RN

Section V

Blueprints for Administration

10

Nursing Administration and the Neuman Systems Model

Dorothy Craig and Charlene Beynon

Nurse administrators in the 1990s are confronted with major new challenges. Mandates for consumer-directed client care, with clients intimately involved in their own health care decision making, and emphases on high-quality, accessible, and cost-effective care to serve diverse client health needs within newly developing patterns of health care delivery have all changed the context of nursing administration.

The Neuman Systems Model has proved its utility for giving direction to nursing administrators in a wide variety of settings, including in-hospital, interdisciplinary, and aggregate community groups. This chapter chronicles the nursing administrative process used in two Canadian health care settings. These concepts and principles should well serve health care administrative systems for diverse populations worldwide.

Betty Neuman

*T*oday's nurse functions in a whirlwind of change. Developments in medical technology, drug therapy, and computer applications have challenged and often changed nursing services. The shrinking of financial resources for health care has also decreased the numbers of professional staff in hospitals and community agencies and, in many cases, has led to increased burdens of responsibility for complex nursing care being carried by fewer nurses.

Nursing administrators are always conscious of the need to ensure that the highest quality of care is provided by their organizations. They are concerned about nurses' ability to deliver that quality of care when they must function within multidisciplinary teams. They are aware that nurses' roles are redefined continually, to keep them relevant to the changing needs of clients and of the health care system. Shorter hospital stays, for example, have increased the level of nursing care required by clients in the community. In some community agencies, nurses have moved from one-to-one contacts with clients to working with groups, aggregates, and entire communities. In many areas, the focus of nursing practice has shifted from treatment to health promotion.

STRATEGIC PLANNING

Strategic planning offers a process by which agencies can gain control over their functions and capitalize on their opportunities. As a "process by which the guiding members of an organization envision its future and develop the necessary procedures and operations to achieve that future," strategic planning asks three basic questions: (a) Where are we going? (b) What is the environment? (c) How do we get there? (Goodstein, Nolan, & Pfeiffer, 1993, p. 3).

The strategic planning process can be empowering. The planning group identifies a vision of the organization's future and develops creative methods to make the vision a reality. The next task is the development of a mission statement that clearly identifies the organization's functions, the client, and the services to be offered. The mission statement ensures that further planning will be based on the agency's purposes and values. To provide guidance for all agency personnel in their daily activities, goals and objectives state clearly the anticipated direction and actions of the organization and the time frames for completion.

Because theory-based nursing practice offers the potential to guide nursing practice in the milieu of change and uncertainty, nursing administrators are supporting the introduction of a conceptual framework for practice. The use of a nursing model can help nurses articulate the scope of their practice both from within and outside of their own profession or agency. Such articulation of practice issues in turn increases the ability of nurse managers and administrators to assess the competence of nursing practice and the quality of nursing care.

Although strategic planning also can be used to *choose* the nursing model most appropriate for the specific agency, initial planning should include staff nurses as well as managers and administrators. The strategic planning questions mentioned earlier can be expanded to include (d) How will the model help us? After an appropriate model has been chosen, goals, objectives, and time frames consistent with the agency's mission statement can be developed.

This chapter presents two examples of implementation of the Neuman Systems Model in diverse settings—a public health agency and a psychiatric facility. The earlier experience of the public health agency provided guidance for the psychiatric facility's implementation project.

MODEL IMPLEMENTATION IN A PUBLIC HEALTH AGENCY

Middlesex–London Public Health Nursing Division

This section describes the experiences of Middlesex–London Health Unit's Public Health Nursing Division in implementing the Neuman Systems Model as the division's framework for nursing practice. Because this implementation was initiated in 1985, the discussion provides a retrospective account of model implementation. The public health agency is a much smaller organization than the psychiatric facility described later in the chapter, and it employs a more homo-geneous staff in terms of educational preparation. As noted in pre-vious publications (Beynon, 1995; Drew, Craig, & Beynon, 1989), this public health nursing division's decision to implement a nurs-ing model in 1985 was precipitated by two external events: the move to theory-based standards by the College of Nurses of Ontario (1990) and the introduction of Standards of Nursing Practice for Community Health Nurses in Ontario (RNAO, 1985).

Choosing the Neuman Systems Model

In 1985, familiarity with nursing models and experience in applying them in daily practice were limited at both the staff and manage-ment levels. Because the standards for community health nurses were based on the Neuman Systems Model, it was selected as the model of choice by the nursing management team. The working group that developed the community health nursing standards found the model especially suited to public health nursing because of (a) its emphasis on the client's perception, with *client* defined as individual, family, group, aggregate, or community; (b) its incorpo-ration of a holistic perspective; and (c) its support of a collaborative approach to practice, which is fundamental to public health nurs-ing (Drew et al., 1989, p. 326). Other factors that encouraged the adoption of the Neuman Systems Model included the Director of Public Health Nursing's experience with the model as a graduate student, the fact that levels of prevention are clearly identified as major concepts within the model, and the model's compatibility with the health unit's mission statement and the nursing division's philosophy.

A decade later, the need for theory-based practice has received greater acceptance, especially among practitioners who have been exposed to nursing models during their undergraduate education or through the literature and through programs for staff development and continuing education. Concurrently, changes in management style have called for partnerships with staff and have emphasized collaboration, collegiality, and shared decision making—concepts perfectly consistent with the values and assumptions inherent in the Neuman Systems Model.

Model Language

We decided to implement the model in its "pure" form, and to avoid modifying less well understood aspects of the model or altering its language, which was perceived as being integral to the model. As staff began to think-through the model, its terminology, regarded initially as a limitation, became more meaningful.

In addition, despite our decision to use the model as a whole, we found that learning activities were initially implementing only selected aspects. We had assumed that gradual implementation would make using the model more manageable. As activities accumulated, however, we acknowledged, and cautioned participants, that it was important not to lose sight of the model as a whole.

Planning the Implementation

We designed a critical path to provide flexibility and direction toward the goals of implementing the Neuman Systems Model and using agency resources with maximum efficiency. In reality, some of the so-called flexibility inherent in the implementation plan resulted from the newness of the venture. (At that time, resources related to theory-based practice in public health settings were scarce, and few role models were available.) The plan evolved under the careful scrutiny of a Steering Committee (Drew et al., 1989). Principles consistent with change theory guided the implementation process. The two key questions were:

1. Why are we doing this?
2. Why are we doing it now?

Planning principles that were incorporated included:

1. Staff and management must share responsibility for implementation of the model.
2. Extensive participation by staff and managers is essential.
3. The project should emphasize the application of the model concepts to practice.
4. The project should encourage independent study and reflection.

5. The importance of both formative and summative evaluation should be stressed.
6. Strategies used to assist participants in learning about the model should be geared to a variety of learning styles.

The implementation process had to be congruent with the model's assumptions, values, and beliefs. Although not explicitly stated at the outset, the principles that guided this initiative—involvement of all partners, shared decision making, an awareness of the internal and external environments, and acknowledgment of strengths—are consistent with the Neuman Systems Model. Reflection suggests that if the project coordinator and the Steering Committee had been more familiar with the Neuman Systems Model, the model could have been used to guide the implementation process. Model concepts could have been used to assess the division's environment and health—for example, the status of the flexible and normal lines of defense or resistance, and the basic structure and stressors. Strategies to implement theory-based practice could have been mutually identified from this assessment and, using the model, their effectiveness could have been evaluated.

Support for Model Implementation

The implementation plan depended on the commitment and work of many individuals. As many nurses as possible were included in the attempt to build a broad base of support and to foster a sense of ownership in the project. The Director of Public Health Nursing's commitment to theory-based practice and support of the implementation plan were fundamental to the success of the project. Among the stressors experienced during the project years were: changes in senior management, relocation, unexpected absences due to illness, and restructuring of the division. Without the Director's commitment and vision, the project—and theory-based practice—would have been abandoned.

Participation by both staff and managers was a critical component of this initiative. The Steering Committee and the staff representatives in each team actively promoted involvement and participation by all partners. (For a complete description of the roles of the Steering

Committee and Neuman representatives, see Drew et al. (1989).) The team supervisors also played a vital role as endorsers of the importance of this initiative. They sanctioned team time for learning activities, functioned as co-learners with their teams, and incorporated the model into their supervisory practice.

Primary responsibility for the project was assumed by the nursing supervisor responsible for staff development and continuing education. Because the project supervisor and the public health nurses and supervisors had to balance their other responsibilities against the demands of this project, it was imperative to use staff time and resources efficiently, to create learning activities that were well planned and reality-based, and to minimize the time spent resolving confusion and uncertainty.

Beyond the existence of committees and the availability of resources to support learning, successful implementation of a theoretical nursing model depends on the willingness of individual staff members to assume responsibility for their own learning and to transform their perspective. As one nurse commented, "[I]mplementing a model should not be divisive . . . in terms of those nurses who are adept with the model and those who are not." Learning must be supported, acknowleded, and shared with others.

Project Goals

Before the project was begun, broad goals for each year of the three-year implementation plan were mapped out by the Steering Committee, composed of both staff and management respresentatives (Drew et al., 1989). The goal for the first year was to have all participants understand the model. Activities to stimulate learning about the model and to highlight its relevance to practice were developed. The second-year goal was to have nurses apply the model in their daily practice. Documentation of the model's use on the nursing record, and employment of the model in case discussions (at team meetings and with the team supervisor) were identified as indicators of this goal. The goal for the third year was to have staff meet the Standards of Nursing Practice for Community Health Nurses in Ontario (RNAO, 1985) by using the Neuman Systems Model as the identified theoretical model for nursing practice.

Time Line

During times of rapid change, it is tempting to delay the implementation of theory-based practice until the environment is more stable and receptive. Today, however, there is no ideal time for such an initiative. Anecdotal experiences indicate that by offering a comprehensive, yet flexible framework for nursing practice, the Neuman Systems Model can assist the practitioner in dealing with a changing and chaotic environment. The model offers a resource to enhance the practitioner's ability to respond effectively to the increased complexity of client concerns. The model can assist the nurse in setting priorities within a caseload—a necessity because of diminishing resources. Because of its utility with individuals, families, groups, and communities, the model can support the nurse in adjusting to the changing role expectations currently being experienced by public health nurses. Such role changes are characterized by an increased emphasis on health promotion and on population-based approaches.

The experiences of this public health nursing division suggest that the following factors should be considered when a time line is developed for the implementation of a nursing model:

1. Identify an end date for completing the project. This is a powerful motivator to ensure that interim goals are achieved and to maintain the energy and momentum needed to sustain the initiative. A specific time frame may also help protect the project and its allocated resources from other competing demands.
2. Allow time at the outset for all participants to express feelings and concerns openly.
3. Acknowledge and, where possible, respond to identified issues.
4. Recognize that it is not feasible for all concerns to be addressed at the outset; some issues will be resolved as the project progresses, and other issues will emerge.
5. Get started with the process and be vigilant; make corrections as needed. Remember that the perfect plan usually can be identified only in retrospect.

6. Be realistic in recognizing other competing demands and priorities intrinsic to a service agency, and adjust the time line accordingly. The time line must be congruent with the unique needs of the setting.

Key Factors for Success

An earlier publication about the experiences of this public health nursing division (Drew et al., 1989) identified the elements that are critical to the successful implementation of a model in practice. A subsequent publication (Beynon, 1995) described the lessons learned about model implementation. The following recommendations are provided as additional guidelines to ensure a successful implementation project:

1. Maintain the momentum and sense of inquiry by routinely integrating opportunities to sustain ongoing commitment to the model and to theory-based practice. Relevant activities might include providing periodic updates, spontaneously using the model to discuss identified practice problems, incorporating the model into staff development programs, circulating a newsletter, and continuing to make resources available.
2. Expand use of the model and develop expertise in areas such as program development and planning, administrative practice, and organizational development.
3. Consult, share experiences, and network with other model users.
4. Allocate staff development funds for purchase of resources and attendance at conferences—for example, the biennial Neuman Systems Model Symposium.
5. Rotate or share responsibility for scanning the literature for new resources and examples of how the Neuman Systems Model is being used in practice, education, administration, and research.

In today's practice environment, characterized by multiple stressors and competing demands, a group or a designated individual should assume a lead role in advocating the use of the model. This task can be done by anybody, or at least somebody, but, regrettably, it may fall to nobody. In this last scenario, not only will the benefits of a successful implementation plan be lost, but, more important, the practice may fail to achieve the degree of excellence that the Neuman Systems Model offers for promoting the health of the population served.

Evaluation

Evaluation of each learning activity was constant throughout the project. Feedback was most helpful, not only for judging the success of the activity, but also for providing direction for future learning activities and for identifying accomplishments. Ongoing dialogue through formative activities was most beneficial in identifying issues requiring follow-up, such as the revision of the nursing record. Similarly, staff completed a survey at the end of each year of the three-year project. Results were useful in identifying both the benefits of using the model (see Beynon, 1995; Drew et al., 1989) and the remaining learning needs.

Frequent and open communication was an essential component of the project. Feedback from the learning activities, responses to submitted questions, and findings from the yearly surveys were shared with teams through their Neuman Representatives (see Beynon, 1995; Drew et al., 1989, for a detailed description) and team supervisors, and through *Neuman Notes,* a publication focused on the model. As part of their role, Neuman Representatives were also expected to identify issues related to model usage within their teams and to share practice stories with other representatives regarding the model's use.

Other approaches were adopted to monitor how effectively the model was being used in practice. They included a review, by the Nursing Audit Committee, of randomly selected discharged clients' records, and use of the model in case discussions between the public health nurse and the assigned supervisor. A review of the discharged clients' records by team supervisors was also effective in monitoring the model's use.

Because many resources were developed by the public health nursing division, the availability of expert clerical support was essential. The project supervisor's clerk also played a major role in collating a resource book that documented the division's experiences in implementing the model.

When practice expectations are changed, especially during times of diminishing resources, it is important to know what value will be added for both the consumer and the practitioner. As described in previous publications (Drew et al., 1989), not all practitioners welcomed the introduction of theory-based practice. Resisters and late adopters made a valuable contribution by asking critical and challenging questions that were instrumental in sharpening the responses to the two key questions: Why are we doing this? and Why are we doing this now? Resisters' scrutiny was helpful in identifying and addressing potential difficulties proactively; however, despite the value of such healthy skepticism, unnecessary delay of the implementation plan is not prudent.

The Nursing Record

Implementation of a model impacts on many areas of practice. The problem-oriented nursing record was compatible with the Neuman Systems Model, but it did not specifically incorporate the model's terminology—an example of where other structures needed to be modified to reflect the model's use. Using a broad-based consultation process, the Records Committee assumed primary responsibility for revising the nursing record. Changes to the record required that the Nursing Audit Tool be revised. In addition, the performance appraisal tool for public health nurses and the division's philosophy statement were modified to reflect more clearly the use of the Neuman Systems Model.

Summary

The success of the implementation project was successful because of the commitment of all levels of nursing personnel in the agency. Participants in the project were able to support one another in learning about the model and using it in practice. They were able to recognize and respect differences in points of view without allowing these differences to impede the goals of the project.

MODEL IMPLEMENTATION IN A PSYCHIATRIC FACILITY

The second example of model implementation occurred at the Whitby Mental Health Center (WMHC) in 1991. This example represents implementation in a large organization that has a mix of nursing services and serves a catchment area of two million people.

Whitby Mental Health Center

The Whitby Mental Health Center, an accredited mental health facility in Ontario, Canada, is funded by the Ontario Ministry of Health. The Center, which first opened its doors in 1919, is one of ten mental health/psychiatric facilities in the province. The Center serves seriously and persistently mentally ill individuals who reside within a large rural and urban catchment area. Comprehensive mental health care is delivered to individuals, families, and groups through a range of multidisciplinary programs offered within inpatient, day treatment, and community outreach settings.

The goals of the Center are: to provide comprehensive treatment and rehabilitation programs to individuals with mental illness, and to assist clients in reintegrating with the community at their most independent level of functioning. The mission statement of the facility includes a belief that each individual has physical, psychosocial, economic, and spiritual needs, and that care for persons should be governed by the principles of availability, accountability, continuity, coordination, and community involvement (Ontario Ministry of Health, 1993).

WMHC employs approximately 400 nursing staff, including both registered nurses (RNs) and registered practical nurses (RPNs). The nurses have formal educational preparation in nursing at the diploma (hospital/community college programs), bachelor's, and master's level (undergraduate/graduate university programs). A large cohort of nurses have a wealth of experience, having practiced in several clinical/community services offered at WMHC and outside the facility.

The philosophy of the nursing department at the hospital is based on the premise that nurses endeavor to maintain and enhance the strengths and coping skills of clients. In-hospital treatment is seen as temporary, goal-directed, and only part of the total consumer care continuum that exists between WMHC and the community it serves, the region of Durham.

HISTORICAL CONSIDERATIONS

Nursing Regulations

The College of Nurses of Ontario (CNO) is the regulatory body for nurses practicing within the province. The mandate of the CNO is to protect the public, and each practicing nurse is required to hold a current Certificate of Competence. In 1990, the CNO released Standards of Nursing Practice, in which four concepts—(a) nursing, (b) person, (c) health, and (d) environment—are used as the foundation for a number of conceptual frameworks, or ways of organizing knowledge and beliefs about nursing. All components of nursing practice can be seen as combinations of or interactions among these basic elements (College of Nurses of Ontario, 1990).

The CNO Standards (1990) served as a catalyst for introducing a nursing conceptual framework to the nursing service at WMHC. Nursing administration, recognizing the merits of integrating theory-based nursing practice, embarked on the challenging journey of model implementation.

Staff Responses

The WMHC prides itself on a history of providing nursing care to mental health consumers for over 75 years. Introduction of a nursing model represented significant change for all members of the hospital culture. Historically, nurses have had limited opportunities to participate in hospitalwide organizational change, such as the implementation of a model to guide nursing practice. Understandably, some nurses were resistant to the idea of introducing something new to a stable and familiar system. "Why fix it if it's not broken?" was a typical objection. Others, candidly reflecting current nursing worklife issues in their reaction to theory-based practice, stated, "We're too stressed . . . overwhelmed . . . ; it's just not the right time to change how we practice." Many nurses, uncertain of the impact that model implementation would have on their individual roles as nurses, asked: "How will this affect my job?" "Does this mean more work for me?" "Will the model change the way I have always practiced?" Staff members, including novice and expert RNs and RPNs, were uncomfortable with their lack of knowledge about nursing theories and how to conceptualize the link between theory and actual practice of the model.

THE CRITICAL PATH TO MODEL IMPLEMENTATION

Resources

Difficult economic times influenced the availability of resources for the model's implementation. From the onset of the implementation project, nursing administrators at the Center strongly supported the shift toward theory-based practice, and they secured financial funding, staff time, and Center services and equipment. In-house nursing staff were asked to serve as key participants in all phases of the project. It was believed that internal members would be familiar with the established nursing work culture and would facilitate acceptance of the model among their peers.

Some uncertainty and resistance to the introduction of a new conceptual framework were anticipated for some nurses. However, the resistance was expected to be reduced if some internal nursing staff were willing to learn about the Neuman Systems Model to nursing practice in the Center. Nurse leaders used the expertise of Neuman Systems Model Trustee members to clarify any difficulties with the model's concepts. Trustee members were also invited to offer nursing staff ongoing opportunities to engage in workshops, forums, and conference presentations.

It was imperative to the success of the project to establish an extensive network of the model's users in hospital, community, and academic settings. Contact with colleagues provided participants at WMHC with opportunities to broaden their knowledge base and share with other practicing nurses clinical experiences of the model's use. Project organizers have attempted to utilize mainly internal resources, but external resources have also been important in creating interest and maintaining enthusiasm about the model.

Choosing the Model

A group of interested nurses met to examine the relevance and utility of several nursing models and to establish a fit between a particular model and the unique nursing culture at WMHC. Nurses from front-line and management positions participated in the selection process. They represented all spheres of nursing service—practice, education, research, and administration.

The Neuman Systems Model was unanimously selected to guide nursing practice. In general, it was believed that the model's theoretical components were congruent with the philosophy, mission statement, goals, and objectives of nursing service within a multidisciplinary team milieu. The model was identified as a framework that would not only support nurses in the shift from traditional nursing care delivery to consumer-centered, hospital, and community-based mental health care, but would also position nursing services to incorporate future initiatives. The fact that the model could provide a framework for nursing care not only to individuals, but also to groups, aggregates, or communities, meant that the model would assist nurses through the anticipated changes in mental health reform that were just beginning at the time of the model's implementation (Ontario Ministry of Health, 1993). The model was viewed as a framework that would help psychiatric nurses in the practice setting to promote realistic, optimal levels of health by creating partnerships with seriously and persistently mentally ill clients (Morris-Coulter et al., 1993).

From the beginning, efforts were made to ground the use of the conceptual framework in the mental health practice setting. Nursing leaders in the implementation project recognized the abstract nature and theoretical complexities that the model presented to practicing nurses. A strategic plan was designed to introduce the model in a systematic, commonsense way to a large group of nurses with varied educational and employment experience (Craig & Morris-Coulter, 1995). Project organizers were sensitive to the fact that most of the nurses had either limited or no previous knowledge of, or experience with, nursing models. To be successful, implementation initiatives had to emphasize learning about the model in ways that were congruent with current nursing practice and were built on existing knowledge bases and clinical expertise. This premise enabled nurses to move gradually from a familiar frame of reference toward incorporation of fundamental assumptions and theoretical concepts of the model into their daily practice.

Historical observation, anecdotal comments, and cues gathered from nurses in practice clearly identified the need for a realistic strategic path. First, an implementation project was developed to introduce all nursing staff to the model. The strategic plan was designed based on the initiatives taken by the Middlesex–London District Health Unit in London, Ontario (Drew et al., 1989). There was evidence that a critical mass of nurses at WMHC were interested in learning more about the model and were eager to engage in change. The plan began to answer the basic who, what, where, when, why, and how of model implementation, and created dialogue among nursing staff. Participation from all levels of staff, during all stages of the project was essential.

Strategic Plan

The implementation project was structured to meet the learning needs and interests of those in the unique nursing culture at WMHC. The project was expected to extend over a three-year period. Selecting the conceptual framework and preparing project staff for theory-based practice were planned as the foci for the first six months; a second six-month period was allotted for orientation of nursing staff to the model; one year was allotted for integrating the model into practice and into multidisciplinary activities; and the final year was designated for maintenance and evaluation.

The decision to implement the model hospitalwide, among all nursing staff, demanded a clearly defined and realistic strategic path. From the beginning, it was important to identify tasks that needed to be performed in all phases of the implementation project, and a host of roles that all nurses at WMHC would be asked to assume. The identification of nurses who could assume significant roles in the project was guided by the Diffusion of Innovations theory, because it was expected that nurses would vary in how long they took to adopt the model. Nurses were seen to be innovators, early adopters, early majority, late majority, or laggards (Rogers, 1983). Innovators served as Steering Committee members and played a vital role in laying the groundwork for the project: selecting the model, establishing the strategic path to guide the project, and making efforts to recruit other nurses into the project.

Steering Committee members represented all spheres of nursing service and provided both global leadership and support for the project within their respective domains. Nursing administration consistently offered support for the mandated implementation project. Neuman Representatives from clinical areas were an essential link in the dissemination of theoretical knowledge and information about experiences with the model in practice. The Representatives' clinical insight helped to focus the activities of the project. Peer networks were established with other practicing nurses. Front-line nurses represented the largest group who engaged in the innovative project at varying levels.

In an effort to introduce more nursing staff to the model, several additional committee structures were formed at the Center level, nursing department level, and clinical/community level. Steering Committee members were convinced that the development of strong collaborative and participatory relationships among nurses would encourage the adoption of new ideas, foster model use, and ultimately enhance the quality of client care (Craig & Morris-Coulter, 1995). Implementation tasks were assigned to each committee according to its particular role in the project. A call for nurses interested in serving as committee members was announced. The benefits of proactively participating in a nursing-driven initiative, as well as the value of the nurses' clinical expertise, were emphasized. Membership was voluntary and was open to nurses from all areas of nursing service. It was emphasized that no previous knowledge of, or experience with, the model was required for those who would serve as committee members. They simply needed an interest in learning about the model and a willingness to share experiences with their nursing peers. Two or three nurses were recruited from each of the 15 clinical/community sites to act as Neuman Representatives, providing a link between front-line practicing nurses and Steering Committee members. A critical mass of about 45 nurses accepted the challenge of implementing the Model in the practice milieu.

Subcommittees

From this collective of interested nurses, subcommittees were formed to focus on three broad areas: (a) promotion, (b) resources, and (c) evaluation. The authors provided a detailed discussion of the subcommittees' structures and purposes, as well as examples of their activities (Craig & Morris-Coulter, 1995). In general, the Promotion Subcommittee initiated a host of activities to raise awareness of, and generate interest in, the model among nurses and hospital personnel. Examples of activities included ongoing special events, newsletters, staff contests, and visual prompts such as bulletin boards, project slogans, and a logo. The committee made an effort to promote the model in friendly, nonthreatening ways that emphasized the benefits of theory-based practice.

The Resource Subcommittee planned a range of educational opportunities that would gradually introduce theoretical components of the model to the large target population of registered nurses and registered practical nurses. An underlying assumption of this focus was a belief that implementation of the model would build on nurses' existing knowledge and that application to practice would be emphasized with experienced nurses in the work setting (Drew et al., 1989). A wide range of activities, including workshops, lectures, and weekly teaching sessions, was provided to encourage a diverse group of adults in the practice setting to learn about the model. Staff were encouraged to choose activities that fit their particular learning style and pace. Efforts were made to interpret the model in ways that were congruent with how mental health nurses were already practicing. Educational events were designed to be easily accessible and nonthreatening.

Practicing nurses seemed most responsive to the use of case studies as a tool for learning about the model. Nurses from each clinical/community area were asked to develop case studies for group discussion. Steering Committee members, who acted as facilitators for the learning sessions, used these case studies to promote staff participation, ownership, and collaboration. In general, case studies provided direction and a structured forum for examining theoretical components of the model. Case studies were tailored to suit the particular subspecialty area, which once again grounded the model in the delivery of client care and encouraged nurses to learn about the model within a familiar context. Among the advantages of using case studies with practicing nurses are opportunities to share perceptions about model concepts, to clarify interpretations, and to examine successful and unsuccessful attempts to use the model in practice. In addition, the participants developed their skills in group process.

The Evaluation Subcommittee was formed to acclimate nurses, from the project's onset, to the importance of critically reviewing the impact of planned change—specifically, the innovation of model implementation. The identified purposes of the evaluation focus were (a) to incorporate mechanisms for evaluating the effectiveness of educational opportunities in promoting nurses' understanding of the theoretical and practical applications of the model, and (b) to examine the impact of model implementation on the delivery of consumer-centered care.

Goals and Objectives

The project's goal was to have all nurses using the Neuman Systems Model as the framework for their practice. Objectives of the project, which were based on experiences shared by professional colleagues in other practice settings, included (a) developing a sense of enthusiasm for learning about the model, (b) promoting an understanding of the theoretical components of the model, and (c) providing opportunities for application of the model in mental health nursing practice (Drew et al., 1989). Although general in nature, the encompassing objectives provided a springboard for specific objectives related to promotion, resources, and evaluation activities (Craig & Morris-Coulter, 1995).

Time Frame

In retrospect, the time lines for the project were adhered to very well. The first phase of the project included planning and orientation to the model. Strategic planning and in-service education sessions for the Steering Committee members and the Neuman Representatives were completed in the first six months. The introduction of the model to the front-line nursing staff through a series of promotion, resource, and evaluation mechanisms was subsequently completed in six months. During this phase, approximately 90% of the total nursing staff complement participated in a 2.5-hour teaching session offered by Steering Committee members in the clinical areas.

Phase Two of the implementation project covered a period of one year. In Phase Two, Neuman Representatives were encouraged to act as resources to peers in their respective clinical/community areas. Front-line nurses from clinical areas began to explore use of the model in their subspecialty. The third year of the project, Phase Three, was identified as a maintenance stage during which increased emphasis would be placed on process and outcome evaluation and on advancing the nurses' understanding of the model in practice. The nursing staff suggested that Phase Three of the project not be concluded at the end of year three; they perceived that integrating the model into practice would be an ongoing challenge. Thus, the project is continuing to grow.

Throughout all phases of the project, the model has been integrated gradually to encompass all aspects of nursing service within a multidisciplinary team framework—for example, client conferences, documentation records, nursing and hospital committee structures, research activities, nursing job descriptions, and performance appraisals.

Key Factors for Success

The following factors emerged as keys to the successful implementation of the model:

1. The pace of the project should be unique to the workplace culture and revised to reflect regular feedback from participants.
2. A supportive network should be established within the agency.
3. A supportive network should be established outside the agency.
4. Both structured and unstructured activities should be used to encourage staff to use the model and critically analyze their practice.
5. Resources that are made available should encourage self-reliance and collegial peer networks.

Evaluation

The evaluation of the model project is often a focus when the project is coming to a close. However, it is essential to consider the evaluative component of the project when the program is being planned. It may be important to collect baseline data before the project gets under way, so that later comparisons can be made.

The evaluation of the project should determine whether the objectives have been met. Thus, it is essential that the objectives be realistic and measurable. Determining at the outset the information that will be required to demonstrate that the objectives have been met will assist staff in establishing an appropriate documentation system for the collection of these data. To ensure that the project adheres to specific target dates, the objectives should also include a time frame for completion.

Both process and outcome objectives should be developed for the project. The process objectives will address how the project will be carried out, and the outcome objectives will address the expected results. Formative evaluation is carried out in the early stages of a project, to determine whether the project is going as planned. Summative evaluation relates to the project's impact (immediate effects) and outcome (long-term effects).

At WMHC, an evaluation focus was included from the start of the project, and staff were socialized to the concept of evaluation. The Evaluation Committee encouraged more process-oriented feedback than outcome-oriented feedback in the early stages of the project. A decision was made to have an outside resource person complete an outcome evaluation for the project. Subsequently, a survey instrument was developed and used to determine the nurses' perceptions of the outcomes of using the Neuman Systems Model in their practice. Focus group meetings were also held at several of the service units, to gain more insight into the nurses' perceptions of the strengths and limitations of using the Neuman Systems Model in their practice. Positive feedback was obtained from both the survey and the focus groups. A majority of the nurses felt that, since they had started to use the model, it had helped them to complete better client assessments, identify client stressors, and work in partnership with clients.

Summary

Many challenges were encountered in this large-scale implementation project. Challenges were heightened by the variation in the staff's formal nursing education, employment experience, and shift schedules, and in the type of nursing care delivery system and the geographical isolation of 15 practice sites. A dynamic program of promotional, resource, and evaluation activities was coordinated to target the diverse variables inherent in a large nursing complement (Craig & Morris-Coulter, 1995).

Many nurses communicated a commitment to the project in their willingness to participate actively in all phases of the project. Risk taking, role modeling, and leadership assumed by many participants facilitated a shift in how the delivery of care was conceptualized. Innovators of the project successfully encouraged a critical mass of interested nurses to "spread the word" about using a model in practice. Maintaining channels of communication within such a large group of participants was at times a challenge, given the complex and demanding nature of the mental health setting. Participants were encouraged to take increased self-responsibility for learning about the model and integrating concepts into their practice. In all, the project was very demanding but worthwhile.

REFERENCES

Beynon, C. E. (1995). Neuman-based experiences in the Middlesex-London Health Unit. In B. Neuman (Ed.), *The Neuman Systems Model* (3rd ed., pp. 537–548). Norwalk, CT: Appleton & Lange.

College of Nurses of Ontario. (1990). *Standards of nursing practice for registered nurses and registered nursing assistants.* Toronto, Canada: Author.

Craig, D. M., & Morris-Coulter, C. (1995). Neuman implementation in a Canadian psychiatric facility. In B. Neuman (Ed.), *The Neuman Systems Model* (3rd ed., pp. 397–406). Norwalk, CT: Appleton & Lange.

Drew, L. L., Craig, D. M., & Beynon, C. E. (1989). The Neuman Systems Model for community health administration and practice: Provinces of Manitoba and Ontario, Canada. In B. Neuman (Ed.), *The Neuman Systems Model* (pp. 315–341). Norwalk, CT: Appleton & Lange.

Goodstein, L. D., Nolan, T. M., & Pfeiffer, J. W. (1993). *Applied strategic planning.* New York: McGraw-Hill.

Morris-Coulter, C., Alder, L., Allan, L., MacDermaid, L., McMullan, J., Peterson, C., & Pritchard, H. (1993). *Partnerships in theory: Implementation of the Neuman Systems Model at an Ontario psychiatric facility.* Poster presented at the Fourth Biennial International Neuman Systems Model Symposium, Rochester, NY.

Ontario Ministry of Health. (1993). *Putting people first.* Toronto, Canada: Author.

Registered Nurses' Association of Ontario (RNAO). (1985). *Standards of nursing practice for community health nurses in Ontario.* Toronto, Canada: Author.

Rogers, E. M. (1983). *Diffusion of innovations* (3rd ed.). New York: Free Press.

ADMINISTRATIVE RESOURCES
OR CONTACTS

United States

Community Nursing Center
University of Rochester
Rochester, NY

Nursing Service
Mercy Catholic Medical Center
Fitzgerald Mercy Division
Darby, PA

Nursing Service
Mt. Sinai Hospital
Hartford, CT

Other Countries

Nursing Service
Elizabeth Breyere Health Center
Tertiary Care
Ottawa, Ontario, Canada

Nursing Services
St. Joseph Hospital
Reykjavik, Iceland

Nursing Service
Jefferson Davis Memorial
    Hospital
Natchez, MS

Nursing Service
Oklahoma State Department of
    Health
Oklahoma City, Oklahoma

Nursing Services
Kuakini Health Care System
Honolulu, Hawaii

Nursing Service
Rykov Hospital
Jonkoping, Sweden

11

Computerization of Self-Care Deficit Nursing Theory in a Medical Center

Jane Bliss-Holtz and Joanne Riggs

I

The work described in this chapter is based on Self-Care Deficit Nursing Theory (S-CDNT), which was developed by Dorothea Orem. Development of a nursing information system based on S-CDNT was begun in 1986 by Nursing Systems International (NSI), with cooperation from Newark Beth Israel Medical Center. This chapter describes implementation of the model in a computerized form in a clinical practice area.

II

The basis of the theory emerges from Orem's observation that some modes of communication and thinking are specific to the discipline of nursing (Orem & Taylor, 1986). Orem's theory of nursing began to evolve from her detailed observations of nurses during her tenure as a nursing consultant for the Division of Hospital and Institutional Services of the Indiana State Board of Health, from 1949 to 1957. The theory was expanded through the work of the Nursing Model Committee of the Catholic University Nursing Faculty in 1965, and the Nursing Development Conference Group in 1968 (Fawcett, 1989; Nursing Development Conference Group, 1973, 1979).

Because the goal of the computerized nursing information system (NIS) was to support nursing practice, using a nursing model as a basis for the information structure seemed a logical choice (Bliss-Holtz, McLaughlin, & Taylor, 1990; Bliss-Holtz, Taylor, & McLaughlin, 1992; Bliss-Holtz, Taylor, McLaughlin, Sayers, & Nickle, 1992; McLaughlin, Taylor, Bliss-Holtz, Sayers, & Nickle, 1990). S-CDNT clearly outlines the operations of nursing practice; therefore, it was chosen as a basis on which to build the NIS.

The concepts of the theory are: Therapeutic Self-Care Demand (TSCD), Self-Care Agency (SCA), and Basic Conditioning Factors (BCFs). The subconcepts are: Universal Self-Care Requisites (USCRs), Developmental Self-Care Requisites (DSCRs), Health Deviation Self-Care Requisites (HDSCRs), Foundational Capabilities and Dispositions (FCDs), Power Components (PCs), and Self-Care Operations (SCOs). These concepts and subconcepts are used in the operations of nursing practice, which are identified by Orem (1991) as: diagnostic, prescriptive, regulatory (including the phases of design, planning, and delivery of care), and control (case management).

The equation that is foundational to practice within the theory is that there is no need for nursing when the Therapeutic Self-Care Demand is equal to the Self-Care Agency. Requisites are defined by Orem (1991) as "formulated and expressed insights about actions that are known to be necessary or hypothesized to have validity in the regulation of aspects of human functioning and development" (p. 121). Therapeutic Self-Care Demand is comprised of three requisites:

1. Universal Self-Care Requisites, which are common to all humans across the life cycle. These include maintenance of the proper intake of air, food, and water.

2. Developmental Self-Care Requisites, which can be of three types: (a) those related to promoting or maintaining development, (b) those related to preventing developmental delays, and (c) those related to mitigating or overcoming existing developmental delays.

3. Health Deviation Self-Care Requisites, which can be in six categories: (a) seeking and securing medical assistance for health care system factors; (b) being aware of and attending to effects and results of health care system factors; (c) carrying out medically prescribed regimes; (d) being aware of, attending to, or regulating effects related to health care system factors; (e) modifying the self-concept in accepting the effects of the health care system factor; and (f) integrating effects of the health care system factor into the lifestyle (Orem, 1991).

Self-Care Agency is composed of Foundational Capabilities and Dispositions (FCDs), Power Components (PCs), and Self-Care Operations (SCOs). Foundational Capabilities and Dispositions (FCDs) are the foundation of all activities of life; the PCs translate the FCDs into actions related to maintaining health and development; the SCOs are the specific actions needed to maintain health and development. Self-Care Operations can be of three forms: (a) estimative (knowing) operations; (b) transitional (decision-making) operations; or (c) productive (action) operations. Basic Conditioning Factors (BCFs) affect both the Therapeutic Self-Care Demand (TSCD) and the Self-Care Agency (SCA) of an individual (Orem, 1991).

Because S-CDNT was introduced previously to the nursing staff at Newark Beth Israel Medical Center as a guide for their practice, use of the NIS was expected to supplement use of the theory by presenting a computerized documentation system that supported theory-based practice in the model.

The structure of the model, and the fit between the model and the practice site, have been described above.

Assumptions underlying the theory include: (a) individuals value their ability to care for themselves without intervention from health care professionals; (b) people are responsible for themselves and tend to seek help when they cannot meet their requisites; (c) the health care system should value people's perspective on their own health; and (d) when health care is needed, the roles of the person and the health care provider should be negotiated and acceptable to both parties (Orem, 1985, 1991).

When implementing the model, a major change in the viewpoint of nurses regarding their role as health care providers may be needed. Members of the nursing profession still persist in assuming primary control of all aspects of an individual's health care, with little input from the client. As implied by the theory, there is a contract between the individual and the nurse in which roles are negotiated. This gives to the individual under health care more power than some nurses are used to conferring.

III

The theory conceptualizes the constant elements and relationships of nursing practice situations (Orem & Taylor, 1986). Because it sets the framework for the operations of nursing practice, it directly relates to guiding nursing practice.

The components of the model that are incorporated into the decision-making process of the NIS are specific to: formulating diagnoses about an *individual's* capabilities for self-care; prescribing the nursing actions relevant to the diagnosed self-care operation limitations of the individual; planning and designing the delivery of the prescribed nursing interventions; and evaluating the effect of the interventions. The model, as used by the NIS, is for supporting and documenting nursing operations specific to individual clients in a wide variety of practice settings across the life span. The model is not being used for documenting nursing practice when groups or communities are considered as the client entities.

The diagnostic decision-making process used in the NIS is based on the concepts described above. Therefore, to employ the system to its full extent, the user should be knowledgeable about the concepts and their relation to each other. In addition, the users need to be knowledgeable about the process by which self-care operation limitation statements are made. These statements are the nursing diagnostic statements that drive the plan of care. Basic knowledge of the concepts and of how the decision-making process operates can be taught in a three-hour class, but true expertise comes with using the model consistently.

The model can be used in a wide variety of nursing practice settings across the life span. Newark Beth Israel Medical Center has been committed to facilitating practice within the model and to developing an NIS that supports the model's use. When theory implementation first began at the medical center, Dr. Dorothy Orem and several experts in use of the model, including Dr. Susan Taylor and Kathy McLaughlin, were consultants to the implementation process. To provide on-site expertise, a nurse educator position was created; its sole purpose was to educate the staff in the concepts of the theory. Currently, that position has been incorporated into the position of the Assistant Director of Nursing—Research and Theory Development. Overseeing the theory-based component of practice and the computer implementation of the model is one of this position's responsibilities.

As mentioned previously, to employ the system to its full extent, the user should be knowledgeable of the concepts of the model. In another area of education, the staff must become familiar with the computerized NIS. Issues such as administrative decisions, users' attitudes toward computer use, and "computer phobia" are common to implementing *any* computerized NIS (Lacey, 1993; Plummer & Warnock-Matheron, 1987; Richards, 1992). Training issues *unique* to use of the theory-based NIS system include: (a) users' familiarity with formulating self-care operation limitation statements (SCOLs) as nursing diagnoses; (b) use of SCOLs to create a plan of care; and (c) use of the care plan for documentation of both the delivery and the effectiveness of nursing interventions.

IV

In the late 1980s, the Vice-President for Nursing, Ruben Fernandez, led the Directors of Nursing in a search for an appropriate theory on which to base nursing practice at Newark Beth Israel Medical Center. In a document written in 1990 as a proposal for the New Jersey Department of Health Nursing Incentive Reimbursement Program, Fernandez and Riggs stated that S-CDNT went "beyond a simple description of nursing tasks to identify and match nursing care resources with individual patient needs within a rigorous, coherent framework" (p. 93). One of the objectives of the proposal was to support development of a computerized NIS that would, in turn, support practice in the model.

As previously mentioned, the nursing staff at Newark Beth Israel Medical Center were knowledgeable about the model. However, one of the problems in implementing it fully was the lack of forms that allowed documentation to occur in a manner that supported the thought processes inherent in the theory. Thus, introduction of a theory-based computerized documentation system was welcomed.

Resources available for this implementation included a grant from the New Jersey Department of Health to implement the computerized model on one of the patient units. Because implementation of this model assumes implementation of an automated patient record, any institution implementing this computerized model should: (a) be firmly committed to implementing a computerized patient record, and (b) recognize the associated costs in terms of hardware, network and mainframe connectivity issues, and staff training prior to committing to the project.

The goal of the implementation of the theory-based computerized NIS was to support and enhance the theory-based practice that already was occurring; thus, there was goal congruence.

The first step was the development of the NIS. A central task was the explication of a decision-making process, based on the model, that would support the type of information processing that was congruent with computer architecture. A database, developed previously under the auspices of Nursing Systems International, relied on groundwork by Dorothea Orem, Susan Taylor, Kathy McLaughlin, and Lynne Nickle, and was created so that a continuous patient record could be generated (Bliss-Holtz, McLaughlin, & Taylor, 1990; Bliss-Holtz, Taylor, & McLaughlin, 1992; Bliss-Holtz, Taylor, McLaughlin, Sayers, & Nickle, 1992). However, the problem of supporting decision-making processes based in the theory had not been well addressed. Consequently, a process that defined the format of a nursing diagnostic statement within the theory and articulated the process of formulating these diagnostic statements was created (Bliss-Holtz, 1995).

Once the decision-making process was explicated and incorporated into a computer program that supported the operations of nursing practice, the planning for clinical implementation of the system began. This process was facilitated by a Nursing Incentive Reimbursement Grant from the New Jersey Department of Health, the goal of which was to improve effective delivery of patient care. Four nursing units were chosen to be monitored for baseline data, which included time spent performing nonnursing tasks and documentation; accuracy and completeness of patient records; and ease of access to patient information. These tasks were performed by Nursing Systems International personnel. One patient unit was chosen as a trial unit for implementation of the computerized NIS.

The next step was planning for and implementing staff education in the decision-making process based in the model and in use of the computerized system. This responsibility was carried by the Assistant Director of Nursing—Research and Theory Development.

As previously mentioned, the majority of the nursing staff had knowledge of the concepts of the model but needed training in the use of the newly derived decision-making process. The wide range of previous computer experience among the nursing staff required tailoring classes to meet various computer skill levels.

Support from the vice president for nursing was important. His role was to find ways to meet the budget needed for system start-up. Costs included local area network (LAN) wiring as well as hardware and software purchases. Cooperation from the medical center's Medical Information System Department was essential because it was decided that all wiring and LAN setup was to be done "in-house," and the necessary personnel resources had to be drawn from and scheduled with this department. The nursing directors' support was key: their budgets supported the extra staffing needed while education regarding the use of the model and the system took place. Support from the Director of Nursing Education and Research was also important. The nurse educators who were to provide educational support to the clinical units reported to this position, so this department's resources would be directly affected. The nurse managers' support was valuable: they were responsible for scheduling and overseeing staff attendance at educational sessions. Finally, staff enthusiasm was key, in that willingness to learn adjunct processes related to the model and to become familiar with a new documentation system would determine the success or failure of the model implementation.

V

The broad aim of the project was to provide theory-based computerized documentation support for the nursing staff in the medical center. Specific objectives, their time lines, and the persons involved in the implementation are given in Figure 11–1.

VI

Examination of the institution's philosophy, for congruence with the underlying assumptions of the model, is recommended. For example, the philosophy of the Department of Nursing at Newark Beth Israel Medical Center states that nurses within the department "recognize that each patient has continuing requirements for self-care and presents to us with varying capacities to meet these needs. Our nursing perspective centers on the provision of quality care which facilitates each patient's optimal self-care ability . . . the patient . . . is entitled to the opportunity of achieving optimal self-care." This philosophy is congruent with the underlying assumptions of the model: individuals value their ability to care for themselves, and nursing functions in a role complementary to the clients' abilities.

Assessment of the nursing staff needs to be made prior to implementation. For the model to be used to its full advantage, nurses must understand the importance of: (a) allowing clients to either perform or oversee as much of their own care as they see fit, (b) providing the environment in which self-care is encouraged, and (c) valuing individuals' perspective of their level of wellness. These philosophical issues have been addressed over a period of years in a variety of in-service education programs, especially those centered around the topic of multicultural aspects of nursing.

Objective	Time Line	Task Assignment
Hardware and software purchase and setup; network wiring for LAN on pilot unit	months 1–5	Vice President for Nursing Assistant Director for Nursing—Research and Theory Development Designated systems administrator
Education/review of the nursing staff (on pilot unit) in the concepts of the model	month 3	Assistant Director for Nursing—Research and Theory Development
Education of the nurse educators in the decision-making process based in the model	month 3	Assistant Director for Nursing—Research and Theory Development
Review/revision of policies and procedures related to use of documentation in the model	months 4–5	Assistant Director of Nursing—Research and Theory Development Director of Nursing Nurse managers Staff nurse committee
Education of the nursing staff (on pilot unit) in use of the decision-making process and computerized system	months 4–5	Assistant Director for Nursing—Research and Theory Development Nurse Educators
Live use of documentation system begins on pilot unit	month 6	Assistant Director for Nursing—Research and Theory Development Nurse educators NSI personnel (systems support)
Evaluation of use of model for: a. comprehensiveness of documentation b. completeness of documentation c. appropriateness of documentation d. timeliness of documentation	month 12	Assistant Director for Nursing—Research and Theory Development Director of Nursing Nurse managers Staff nurse committee

Figure 11–1. Objectives, Time-Line, and Assignment of Tasks for Implementing Theory-Based Computer Support.

As previously mentioned, it is difficult to separate issues related to implementing theory-related practice from issues relating to implementing a computerized documentation system, because the two are so intimately intertwined in this example. Although associated more with computerized documentation, the institution's commitment to the resources needed for computerized implementation is essential. The costs associated with hardware, software, LAN setup, technical support, and staff training need to be carefully considered. If the sole motivation of computerizing documentation is supporting the model, then it is a costly solution. If, however, the institution is considering implementing computerized documentation in any case, these costs will be present whether this model of decision making is implemented concurrently or not.

It is strongly recommended that, at a minimum, a consultant is available who has a deep knowledge of and experience in teaching others to implement the theory. The department of nursing at Newark Beth Israel Medical Center had access not only to Dorothea Orem's sound advice, but also to the advice of several experts in the theory. The Department of Nursing's commitment also was demonstrated when a position was added, with the major objective of supporting staff in their learning and practice of the theory. This addition occurred several years prior to implementing the computerized model.

Commitment to the theory-based computerized documentation system also means that the nursing department must be willing to reexamine policies and procedures related to how nursing documentation is to be performed. For example, the nursing care plan produced by the system is in two parts: (a) a list of self-care operation limitations specific to the client, and (b) a list of related helping methods, or interventions, that need to be performed to resolve those limitations. Policies and procedures related to the timely updating and evaluating of these care plans need to be considered in light of the ease with which they can be revised electronically. Another issue is: What hard copy reports are acceptable, not only to the nursing department, but also to the medical record requirements of the institution? It is wise to share with other departments maximum information as to the possible impact of theory-based documentation. A central issue that often emerges in interdisciplinary discussions is fear that nursing will speak a language that other health care disciplines will not understand. Because most disciplines understand the concept of patient deficit, even if not in the same form that the model addresses, apprehension quickly is laid to rest.

The integrity of the decision-making model in the computerized system was addressed through validation by experts in the theory, who ensured that the process was consistent with the concepts and theoretical propositions of the model.

Evaluation of the nursing staff (for their understanding of the theory) and of the nurse educators (for their ability to teach the theory) is being performed through evaluation of theory-based competencies, which were developed by the Division of Nursing Standards Assurance and Research (Bliss-Holtz & Riggs, 1994). Evaluation of the nursing staff for use of the computerized documentation system will be addressed by measuring: (a) comprehensiveness of documentation, (b) completeness of documentation, (c) appropriateness of documentation, and (d) timeliness of documentation six months after initial use of the theory-based system.

Newark Beth Israel is the first health care facility to use this patient documentation system.

REFERENCES

Bliss-Holtz, J. (1995). *Theory-related nursing diagnoses: A process generated from Self-Care Deficit Nursing Theory.* Manuscript submitted for publication.

Bliss-Holtz, J., McLaughlin, K., & Taylor, S. (1990). Validating nursing theory for use within a computerized nursing information system. *Advances in Nursing Science, 13*(2), 46–52.

Bliss-Holtz, J., & Riggs, J. (1994). Competency-based assessment of theory-based practice. *International Orem Society Newsletter, 2*(3), 6–7.

Bliss-Holtz, J., Taylor, S., & McLaughlin, K. (1992). Nursing theory as a base for a computerized nursing information system. *Nursing Science Quarterly, 5*(3), 124–128.

Bliss-Holtz, J., Taylor, S. G., McLaughlin, K., Sayers, P., & Nickle, L. (1992). Development of a computerized information system based on Self-Care Deficit Nursing Theory. In J. Arnold & G. Pearson (Eds.). *Computer applications in nursing education and practice* (pp. 87–93). New York: NLN Press.

Fawcett, J. (1989). *Analysis and evaluation of conceptual models in nursing* (2nd ed.). Philadelphia: Davis.

Fernandez, R., & Riggs, J. (1990). *Proposal for work redesign and the implementation of computer support of theory-based practice.* Trenton: New Jersey State Department of Health.

Lacey, D. (1993). Nurses' attitude towards computerization: A review of the literature. *Journal of Nursing Management,* 239-243.

McLaughlin, K., Taylor, S., Bliss-Holtz, J., Sayers, P., & Nickle, L. (1990). Shaping the future: The marriage of nursing theory and informatics. *Computers in Nursing, 8*(4), 174-179.

Nursing Development Conference Group. (1973). *Concept formalization in nursing. Process and product.* Boston: Little, Brown.

Nursing Development Conference Group. (1979). *Concept formalization in nursing. Process and product* (2nd ed.). Boston: Little, Brown.

Orem, D. E. (1985). *Nursing: Concepts of practice* (3rd ed.). New York: McGraw-Hill.

Orem, D. E. (1991). *Nursing: Concepts of practice* (4th ed.). St. Louis: Mosby.

Orem, D. E., & Taylor, S. (1986). Orem's general theory of nursing. In P. Winstead-Fry (Ed.), *Case studies in nursing theory* (pp. 37-71). New York: National League for Nursing.

Plummer, C., & Warnock-Matheron, A. (1987). Training nursing staff in the use of a computerized hospital information system. *Computers in Nursing, 5,* 6-9.

Richards, J. (1992). Implementing a computer system: Issues for nurse administrators. *Computers in Nursing, 10,* 9-13.

Section VI

International Blueprint Application

12

The Roper–Logan–Tierney Model: A Model in Nursing Practice

Nancy Roper, Winifred Logan, and Alison Tierney

INTRODUCTION: USING A MODEL IN PRACTICE

Often described as the "Activities of Living" model for nursing, the Roper-Logan-Tierney Model was first published in *The Elements of Nursing* in 1980 and is generally regarded as the first British model for nursing. It has become well known over the years and, although originally envisaged as a conceptual framework to assist beginning nursing students, the model has been used widely as a conceptual framework for nursing practice in a range of settings. It has been

289

utilized in several other countries, including Finland, Italy, Portugal, and India.

The specific implementation of the Roper–Logan–Tierney Model that is described here comes from Manchester, England, where a nurse teacher, Sue Whittam, along with colleagues, used the model to guide practice, first in one ward, then throughout the hospital, then throughout wards and departments in an entire National Health Service Trust (a group of hospitals and services). We are indebted to Sue Whittam for providing detailed information about this specific implementation of the model, and we draw on her input throughout the chapter.

The Manchester project arose out of Whittam's concern about the theory–practice gap that exists in individualized care planning. As a nurse teacher, she had identified that basic nursing students—relative novices—could in fact apply the concepts of nursing models to patient care with relative success. Yet, in clinical areas, where experts are responsible and accountable for nursing practice, there was less evidence that models were influencing practice. The students were confused, and Whittam felt that her credibility as a nurse and as a teacher was under threat.

What initially was a personal quest developed into a more general search to see whether models could improve standards of nursing practice. And if not, what might be the alternatives?

Whittam's ideas became more focused when, as part of a degree studies program, she chose an assignment that involved devising a plan for using the Roper–Logan–Tierney model in a practice setting. From the related review of literature, she realized, among other things, that standards of care planning were very much under the microscope, particularly from the UK's Department of Health, the UK Audit Commission, and the UK Central Council (the professional registering body). In effect, these organizations were pointing to evidence of "fragmented" nursing that lacked theoretical underpinnings. Concurrently, nurse managers were concerned about a real theory–practice–management gap. When Whittam offered her carefully considered theoretical plan as a possible means of reducing the gap, the suggestion was met with some enthusiasm. The climate for change seemed right.

The project required considerable initial preparation, personally and with interested colleagues. To assist with planning, the theory-practice-theory approach described by Marriner-Tomey (1989) was used. Eventually, it was decided to initiate the project in a female surgical ward where staff had already expressed a keen interest in developing their nursing practice. A series of time-consuming and challenging activities were undertaken—questionnaires; audits; assessment and care planning guidelines; meetings; and preparation of teaching materials. Importantly, however, good working relationships and shared vision existed among clinicians, managers, and educationalists across all health care disciplines.

After Whittam and her colleagues agreed that they would use the Roper-Logan-Tierney model, she contacted the authors and invited discussion and feedback.

So far, the findings from the project reveal that, following initial preparation, one of the best ways for the model to begin to influence care delivery is to integrate the concepts of the model into nursing documentation. By systematically applying the concepts to every stage of the nursing process, the "thinking" can begin to influence the practice. According to Whittam, the documents also acted as a teaching tool.

Preparing documentation sounds easy, but at least four drafts of a "Patient's Nursing Record" based on the Roper-Logan-Tierney model were painstakingly produced, reviewed, and revised before an acceptable document could be finalized and utilized. The current version is now being monitored for a year.

The implementation of the model is discussed later in this chapter. Let us first briefly describe and discuss the Roper-Logan-Tierney model.

EVOLUTION OF THE ROPER–LOGAN–TIERNEY MODEL

We believe a model for nursing is essentially a conceptual framework. Models help nurses to interpret the theory that underpins nursing practice by identifying key concepts and indicating relationships between the concepts. Models act as a growing point for further thinking about the discipline. A model may be expanded or changed—or indeed, may be discarded if it is no longer useful and no longer reflects the reality of everyday practice.

Attempts to identify the knowledge base of nursing practice were pioneered by our North American colleagues at least two decades before nurses in the UK began to make a contribution to theoretical thinking. Perhaps this is because North Americans were 50 years ahead of Europeans in establishing nursing programs in a university setting, a milieu where research and the search for knowledge are expected. The first North American basic nursing program was offered in an academic setting in Minnesota in 1909. In Europe, the first one was offered at the University of Edinburgh in 1960. (It is perhaps no coincidence that Roper, Logan and Tierney are all graduates of that university.)

Prior to our collective work, the original Roper model was published in 1976 as a research monograph, "Clinical Experiences in Nursing Education." This early model was an extrapolation from an extensive literature review related to a possible core of nursing, and also from the project's findings about students' experiences of nursing in a general, a psychiatric, and a maternity hospital, and in twelve community nursing settings.

The original Roper model was expanded and revised to produce the Roper-Logan-Tierney model, and the result of this work was first published in 1980 as *The Elements of Nursing.* Ongoing refinements have been made, and the latest version of the model is described in the 4th edition of *The Elements of Nursing,* to be published in 1996.

In an attempt to show how the first version of our model could be used as a conceptual framework for the process of nursing, *Learning to Use the Process of Nursing* was published in 1981.

Using a Model for Nursing, published in 1983, describes a project we set up to test our belief that the model is a conceptual framework that can be used in a variety of nursing settings. The project involved real patients/clients, and the nursing studies were carried out and written up by practicing nurses who worked with us on this project.

The exercises and feedback we have received from numerous people who have subsequently used or analyzed the model have resulted in our current presentation. Models are not made up of a few transient thoughts hastily put together; they are developed carefully and systematically, sometimes as a result of research, and may involve months or years of observing nursing practices and thinking about *why,* as well as *how* nursing is carried out. The process of refinement is ongoing. To paraphrase Meleis's (1985) comment about books, we could say, "A model is never complete because ideas are never complete."

THE ROPER–LOGAN–TIERNEY MODEL

The Roper-Logan-Tierney model for nursing is based on a model of living. Each model has five components:

Model of Living	*Model for Nursing*
1. Twelve Activities of Living (ALs)	1. Twelve Activities of Living (ALs)
2. Life span	2. Life span
3. Dependence/Independence continuum	3. Dependence/Independence continuum
4. Factors influencing the ALs: biological psychological sociocultural environmental politicoeconomic	4. Factors influencing the ALs: biological psychological sociocultural environmental politicoeconomic
5. Individuality in living	5. Individualizing nursing

The first four components have the same wording in both models. In each model, the unique mix of the first four components, for any individual, contributes to the fifth component: individuality in living, in the model of living, and individualizing nursing, in the model for nursing. It will be readily agreed that individualizing nursing can only be accomplished if the nurse knows something about the person's individuality in living.

Activities of Living (ALs)

The Activities of Living (rather than activities of *daily* living, for they are not all daily) are the focus of our model (Figures 12–1 and

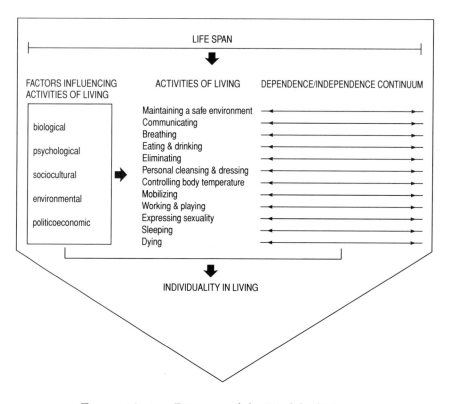

Figure 12–1. Diagram of the Model of Living.

12-2) because they are central to our view of nursing. We believe
that nursing is concerned with:

> *helping people to prevent; alleviate or solve; or cope with those
> problems related to Activities of Living which are amenable to
> nursing.*

In using the term "problems," we are not focusing only on *actual*
problems. The concept of *potential problems* permits the model to
apply to promotion and maintenance of health, and to participation
in a screening program. We exploit the concept of potential problems also to highlight the preventive nature of nursing; the concept
identifies the necessity for health education and the important role

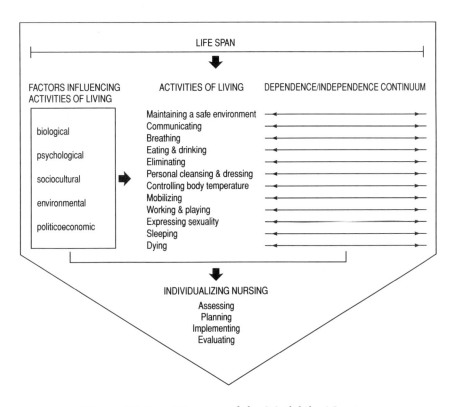

Figure 12–2.   Diagram of the Model for Nursing.

of health teaching even in an illness setting such as a hospital—for example, in preventing deep venous thrombosis postsurgery with a possible consequence of pulmonary embolism.

We deliberately chose to use the concept of Activities of Living rather than basic human needs, which has been widely used in nursing. An example is Maslow's categorization of needs (based on his theory of motivation), arranged in order of priority and creating a "hierarchy" that is frequently represented by a pyramid. The important point here is that, unlike needs, ALs have an advantage for a nursing model in that they are observable and can be explicitly described and in some instances objectively measured. And nursing research is concerned with increasing the availability of appropriate tools for measuring patient/client behavior and outcomes.

The terms we chose as name for the twelve ALs also merit comment; finding suitable names for some of the ALs was difficult! We deliberately decided to use words that would be readily comprehensible to both nurses and patients/clients. In so doing, we chose to be consistent in emphasizing their active nature (hence, eliminat*ing* rather than eliminat*ion*), and we attempted to be comprehensive. "Washing and dressing" is the more commonly used term, but we decided on "personal cleansing and dressing" because it is all-embracing of the various activities subsumed in that AL—care of the skin, perineum, hair, nails, and teeth. It is interesting to reflect that, in the early years of our work on the model, use of the term "expressing sexuality" raised many eyebrows. We explained in the text how it applied not only to the narrow interpretation of "sexual function" but to a much wider concept of expressing femininity/masculinity. Now, however, all aspects of sexuality are discussed freely in the media, and the term "expressing sexuality" has become commonly used by nurses. Similarly, using the term "dying" was questioned initially because not many basic nursing texts discuss this subject in any detail, in terms of either the dying person's reaction, or the grief and bereavement of family members and friends. This topic also has lost some of its taboo.

As a consequence, although some of the names seemed rather unusual when *The Elements of Nursing* was first published, we were adamant about using our deliberately and carefully chosen terms for the twelve ALs, and we have retained them:

1. Maintaining a safe environment
2. Communicating
3. Breathing
4. Eating and drinking
5. Eliminating
6. Personal cleansing and dressing
7. Controlling body temperature
8. Mobilizing
9. Working and playing
10. Expressing sexuality

11. Sleeping

12. Dying

Although each AL appears to be simple, with some thought, its *complexity* becomes obvious. In addition, the ALs are *closely related* and interactive. When obtaining information at an initial assessment about one AL, the nurse is likely to find out a great deal about other ALs. For instance, discussion of eating and drinking could lead the person to mention eliminating habits. And a problem with one AL may well cause problems with one or more of the others; for example, a problem with mobilizing is likely to influence the ALs of eliminating; personal cleansing and dressing; and working and playing. The close relationship between and among the ALs is reiterated in all of our discussion of the model.

So, too, is another aspect of ALs: there are *priorities* among them, and they change according to circumstance. This notion is particularly important for nursing. For example, immediately after a myocardial infarction, the AL of expressing sexuality will have a low priority; but quite quickly, the person is usually concerned about his or her general appearance and, before discharge from the hospital, the patient may want to know whether, and when, it will be safe to resume sexual relations. On the other hand, for a woman having elective surgery for mastectomy, many aspects of that same AL will be important even on admission, as well as throughout the pre- and postoperative periods, and in the long term. Our accounts of the model emphasize that different circumstances create different priorities and, therefore, common sense and professional judgment must be applied by nurses in making decisions about the relative priorities of the ALs.

Closely associated with the order of priority among ALs is the notion of *relevance*. Although the twelve ALs are relevant to nursing, not all of them are necessarily relevant to any one patient/client all of the time. Any one AL, or indeed several ALs, may receive consideration but not require documentation at all, or may merit documentation only at certain points in a client's nursing plan. With the advent of increasingly short-stay hospital admissions, the notion of relevance is particularly cogent.

Life Span

It is not difficult to accept life span as another key component of the model. Some models are built around theories of growth and development; ours incorporates this dimension. "Living" is concerned with the whole of a person's life, and each person has a life span, however long or short. It begins at birth, the event that heralds "living" separately from the mother, and it ends at death. There is only one direction of movement along the life span.

Even in everyday language, the various life stages are described as infancy, childhood, adolescence, adulthood, and old age. Each of these stages is characterized by biological, intellectual, emotional, and social developments. In the early years, some of these developments result in increased independence in particular ALs. Age, the fact that identifies the stage on the life span, is the criterion for acquisition of independence in ALs such as eating and drinking, personal cleansing and dressing, and mobilizing.

The life span component of the model serves as a reminder that nursing is concerned with people of all ages; an individual may require nursing at any stage in the life span. Nurses still use the terms maternity nursing, pediatric nursing, nursing of adults, nursing the elderly, and so on. Jourard (1972) maintained that:

> these are convenient labels describing the place where the given nurse works, and broad categories into which the patient may be assigned . . . [they encourage] a kind of unhelpful confusion in thinking, teaching and practice . . . they mask something basic which all branches of nursing share.

Taking account of a person's age has always been recognized as important in nursing, but we have probably failed to verbalize the ways in which it is important. It influences all phases of the process of nursing—assessing, planning, implementing, and evaluating— and is an essential consideration in individualizing nursing. Two patients may have the same problem with an AL, but the fact that one patient is 25 and the other is 85 may mean that different goals are appropriate. Age can influence selection of a nursing intervention for the same problem; medication dosage is an obvious example.

Similarly, the appropriate diet for a small child will be different from that for a young adult, and different again for an elderly person. The life span component of our model addresses these issues.

Dependence/Independence Continuum

The third component of the model is a dependence/independence continuum, with total dependence and total independence at the two poles. We wrestled with this concept for some time; indeed, we asked ourselves whether a state of total independence actually existed. Finally, we decided that, in a nursing context, the concepts of dependence and independence are only meaningful as relative terms; hence these ideas are presented by means of a *continuum* along which there can be movement in either direction, according to circumstance. We maintain that the concept of dependence/independence applied in general to a person is too global to be meaningful, but attaching it to each AL helps to give it meaning. In Figures 12–1 and 12–2, a continuum appears alongside each AL; its arrows indicate that status can change in either direction, a most important determinant of nursing the individual person. Unlike other nursing models (Orem's, for example) that emphasize the attribute of self-care, ours accommodates the notion that dependence can be an inevitable and acceptable state.

Relating the dependence/independence status of people at different stages of the life span illustrates the close link between these two components of the model. However, not all people are born with the potential to become independent in all twelve ALs as they progress along the life span. For example, for those who are severely mentally and/or physically disabled, whether at home or in an institutional setting, the goal should be acquisition of optimal independence for each AL.

At a later stage in the life span, there are people who, having gained independence in the ALs, may be deprived of it by circumstances such as accident or disease. In these instances, the goal will be to regain as much independence as possible for the affected ALs. This goal can only be achieved by individualizing the nursing contribution to the total rehabilitation program devised by the multidisciplinary health team.

In this age of high technology, one needs no reminder that many gadgets and appliances are available to help those with a congenital or acquired disability to achieve, maintain, or regain independence or a form of "aided independence" in particular ALs, and this is an important dimension within our concept of dependence/independence.

It is absolutely essential that nursing records contain adequate detail about a person's dependence/independence status for each AL—that is, exactly what can and cannot be done independently—and any previous coping mechanisms. (These items appear on our Patient Assessment Form, offered as a guideline, and will be mentioned later.) There is of course a fine dividing line between depriving a patient of independence of which he or she is capable, and leaving a patient to be independent when he or she is incapable. Helping the patient to accept dependence when this is necessary—perhaps transiently, perhaps permanently—is part of the skill of professional judgment.

Factors Influencing the ALs

So far, three components of the model have been mentioned: the ALs, the life span, and the dependence/independence continuum. Although everyone carries out ALs at every stage of the life span with varying degrees of independence, each person does so differently. To a large extent, these differences arise because *a variety of factors influence the way a person carries out ALs.* These factors form the fourth component of the model.

In the model of living, this component explains why there are individual differences in the way the ALs are carried out. Those selected for discussion in our model for nursing are mentioned because of their relevance to nursing or because they provide a context for the discussion of nursing.

It would be possible to devise a long list of different kinds of factors: biological; intellectual and emotional; social, religious, spiritual, cultural, philosophical, ethical; environmental; political, economic, and legal. For the purposes of our model, however, factors are grouped into five categories:

1. Biological
2. Psychological
3. Sociocultural (including religious, spiritual, and ethical)
4. Environmental
5. Politicoeconomic (including legal).

Deliberately, these factors are focused on each Al separately (see Figures 12-1 and 12-2). It would be possible to focus them on the individual as a total entity, discussing in general terms the effects of the five groups of factors on life style. But this approach is too global. Instead, discussing them as they influence each of the twelve ALs highlights the individuality in living.

The five factors, as well as being related to the other components of the model, are themselves interrelated. In fact, when assessing a patient/client, it may be difficult to make a clear-cut distinction between the influence of biological as against psychological factors, or between sociological and politicoeconomic factors. Despite the overlap, we discuss the five factors separately in *The Elements of Nursing,* and as each nurse becomes familiar with the thinking behind our model, it becomes possible to amalgamate data about a client into relevant and manageable categories for the purposes of recording.

The five factors draw on theory from subjects that are disciplines in their own right (for example, biological sciences, arts, and social sciences) and are studied in separate parts of a basic nursing curriculum. The nurse has to integrate relevant concepts from these disciplines into each AL in the model and apply them in nursing practice.

Individuality in Living

In each individual, the unique mix of the first four components leads to the fifth component, individuality in living. Individuality can manifest itself in many different ways:

- How a person carries out the AL.
- How often the person carries out the AL.

- Where the person carries out the AL.
- Why the person carries out the AL in a particular way.
- What the person knows about the AL.
- The attitude the person has toward the AL.

Our model is based on the individual. However, within a family, an individual functions in relation to the individuality of other members of the family (or the group inhabiting a household), and it may be important for the nurse to understand the individuality of other family members when helping the person who has contacted the health service.

Individualizing Nursing

Knowledge of a person's individuality in living is, in our view, an essential prerequisite to individualizing nursing. What we mean by individualizing nursing (Figure 12-2) is accomplished by using the process of nursing (or whatever equivalent term is used) in relation to the concepts of our model and involves:

- Assessing.
- Planning.
- Implementing.
- Evaluating.

Our rationale for incorporating the "process" in our model is to reinforce the relationship between the process and the conceptual framework.

Overemphasis on nursing process documentation is to be avoided; on the other hand, it is pertinent to recognize that some method has to be chosen to record data so that all members of staff can read it easily and coordinate their efforts for the benefit of the client.

Assumptions on Which the Model Is Based

The selected concepts and the relationships among the concepts in a nursing model are means of interpreting the discipline of nursing. It is not surprising, therefore, that creators of models give considerable attention to the assumptions that underlie their approach to the discipline. Fawcett (1984) considered that creators of models for nursing should make their assumptions explicit because they are indicative of the authors' values and their special points of emphasis. The authors of the Roper–Logan–Tierney model make the following assumptions:

- Living can be described as an amalgam of Activities of Living (ALs).
- The way ALs are carried out by each person contributes to individuality in living.
- The individual is valued at all stages of the life span.
- Throughout the life span until adulthood, the individual tends to become increasingly independent in the ALs.
- Independence in the ALs is valued, but dependence should not diminish the dignity of the individual.
- An individual's knowledge, attitudes, and behavior related to the ALs are influenced by a variety of factors, which can be categorized broadly as biological, psychological, sociocultural, environmental, and politicoeconomic.
- The way in which an individual carries out the ALs can fluctuate within a range of normal for that person.
- When an individual is "ill," there may be problems (actual or potential) with the ALs.
- During the life span, most individuals experience significant life events that can affect the way they carry out ALs, and may lead to problems, actual or potential.
- The concept of potential problems incorporates the promotion and maintenance of health and the prevention of disease; it also identifies the role of the nurse as a health teacher, even in illness settings.
- Within a health care context, nurses work in partnership with the client/patient who, except for special circumstances, is an autonomous, decision-making person.

- Nurses are part of a multiprofessional health care team who work in partnership for the benefit of the client/patient and for the health of the community.
- The specific function of nursing is to assist the individual to prevent, alleviate or solve, or cope with problems (actual or potential) related to the ALs.

Relationship with Metaparadigm Concepts

In 1977, Kuhn coined the term "metaparadigm" to describe the global concepts of a discipline. Despite apparent differences in models for nursing, there is now considerable agreement (Fawcett, 1978; Flaskarud & Halloran, 1980) that the global concepts common to most models are:

- Person.
- Environment.
- Health.
- Nursing.

The Roper-Logan-Tierney model was not deliberately constructed around this metaparadigm—in fact, it predated the articulation of this idea—but it does address all four of these concepts.

We do not see the various models for nursing as competitors. Model builders are attempting to identify the core of nursing, which we regard as a collaborative exercise. Perhaps the quest can be summed up as:

Thus the task is, not so much to see what no one has seen yet; but to think what nobody as thought yet, about what everybody sees.
—Schopenhauer

APPLICABILITY OF THE MODEL IN THE PRACTICE SETTING

The model was originally designed to try to articulate the "core" of nursing. Irrespective of the setting where nurses work, it was thought, there is a common base of knowledge and theory. To quote Reilly (1975):

> *We all have a private image (concept) of nursing practice. In turn this private image influences our interpretation of data, our decisions and our actions. But can a discipline continue to develop when its members hold so many differing private images? The proponents of conceptual models of practice are seeking to make us aware of private images, so that we can begin to identify commonalities in our perception of the nature of practice.*

We believe that, irrespective of the nursing specialty, the core is basic and the different aspects of our model can be emphasized to suit the circumstances of the specialty in relation to life span, dependence/independence, and factors (biological, psychological, sociocultural, environmental, politicoeconomic) insofar as they affect the individual's Activities of Living. The model could be adapted to community nursing, pediatric nursing, care of the elderly, psychiatric nursing, intensive care, and so on.

Having identified what *seemed* to be a core of nursing, the original model was intended to provide a framework in which students would learn about the art of nursing.

GENERAL APPLICATION OF THE MODEL

Our original version of the model was tried out in a variety of clinical settings as described in *Using a model for nursing* (1983). A more recent version of the model has been used by Jamieson, McCall, and Blythe (1992). Currently, the model is known to be used as a basis for guiding, directing, teaching, and evaluating in a number of practice settings in the UK, and we have selected the Manchester project, as explained earlier, to provide an example of a recent application.

At the end of a paper presented in London, at the First National Conference for Nurse Education and Practice, in 1994, a summarization of the benefits observed in the Manchester project are as follows:

- Patients are receiving more purposeful assessment and real problem identification, and have a greater chance of individualized care.
- Practitioners have developed knowledge, skills, and attitudes regarding the value of nursing models and can relate these attributes to job satisfaction, responsibility, and accountability.
- Students are able to experience the links between theory and practice and to maximize "reflective practice" in order to develop the knowledge, skills, and attitudes required in nursing.
- Educators have increased their competency and credibility to teach theory by developing their awareness about the realities of nursing practice; therefore, they are able to appreciate the important part they play in contributing to standards of nursing.
- Managers have increased their awareness of the realities of planning and delivering patient care; and of their responsibilities toward resource management and staff development.

Intended Patient/Client Populations

The model focuses on individuals because individualizing nursing can be possible only if nurses appreciate the person's individuality in living (Figure 12–1).

But individuals do not live in isolation. Most people are part of a family (or a variation of group living), and the individuality of other members of the group may influence the person who is seeking nursing advice or help. It may be necessary for the nurse to consider the behavior/circumstances of these "others" (their individuality) in order to plan nursing for an individual.

"Simplicity" of the Model

The model is *apparently* simple; more or less, it is couched in everyday language. But it is not simplistic; indeed, the concepts are complex. Whittam indicated that its use in practice depends on how well the model has been studied and understood by its implementers. To pluck out only one concept (e.g., the ALs), as has been done in some instances without utilizing the other concepts, does not allow adaptability to different practice settings. When this occurs, potential users, besides being frustrated by what seem to be the model's inadequacies, lose the opportunity offered by the model to underpin practice.

COSTS OF IMPLEMENTATION

To cover costs, many centers in the UK that have used our model have had to implement it using available resources, which is certainly challenging and not always conducive to success.

Person time is needed by the initiators for thinking and reflecting and for devising activities to promote successful implementation of any nursing model. Considerable time is also needed for staff meetings, and the time involved (although "hidden") does mean financial cost. More tangible costs can be assessed in relation to the preparation of (a) relevant documents for nursing records that reflect the model, and (b) teaching packages about the model.

In addition, intensive educational and managerial support is imperative throughout the lengthy period during which implementation, monitoring, and evaluation proceed. Changes were of crucial importance to success in the Manchester project, and staff time costs money, although it was not specifically calculated.

Whittam provided some costings for the Manchester project but admitted that they are only estimates. However, she intends to monitor the financial implications more closely when another interested NHS Trust Group invites her methods of implementation. Hopefully, some of the inevitable problems encountered by an innovator will be bypassed! Nevertheless, she emphasizes that, quite apart from financial costs, much goodwill on the part of many implementers has made it difficult to determine the actual sums of money involved; the implementers have given freely of their time.

IMPLEMENTATION OF THE MODEL

Assessment of the Setting

For Sue Whittam, the climate was right for change in 1993. At the national level, concern was being voiced about the need for better integration of theory and practice in British nursing; and the UKCC

(United Kingdom Central Council for Nursing, Midwifery, and Health Visiting) had issued guidance on Standards for Records and Record Keeping. At the local level, nurse managers who are responsible for nursing practice in hospital and community settings, and who are also involved with the education of nursing students (most service settings in the UK provide practice experience for student nurses), were recognizing that there was a continuing theory-practice-management gap. They also recognized that national bodies, as mentioned above, were demanding action.

Planning for Implementation of the Model

The initiators of the Manchester project searched the literature on nursing models and, in addition, made inquiries about current care planning practices.

A *Care Planning Questionnaire* was designed to ascertain the level of knowledge and skills, and the attitudes toward current care planning practices. The recipient nurses were told that the initiators were seeking their guidance in preparation for improvements in care planning. Various questions were asked, to ascertain, for example:

- Which nursing model was used to guide practice and how well it was understood.
- Whether the model matched the needs of patients/clients in that setting.
- Whether nursing students had more or less knowledge about models for nursing than qualified staff.
- Whether models were perceived as being only for educational purposes or were also useful in practice.
- What degree of interest was directed toward developing/improving the current system.
- Whether there were any identifiable factors that prevented the nursing staff from delivering good standards of care.

A *Care Plan Audit* was also conducted, to gain knowledge about current care plans. The following are samples of questions:

- Is there a ward philosophy that reflects/recognizes individualized patient care?
- Do care plans reflect a nursing model?
- Are patients' records kept securely and is confidentiality ensured?
- Does patient assessment reflect the individual needs of the patient (biological, psychological, sociocultural, spiritual, and economic aspects)?
- Do care plans demonstrate a problem-solving approach?
- Are problems patient-centered?
- Do care plans address planning for discharge?
- Do care plans accurately identify care requirements by nurses and other health professionals?
- Do care plans provide an accurate baseline against which improvements (or other developments) can be measured?
- Does the primary nurse discuss the plan with the patient/family?
- Do care plans show evidence of patient/family involvement?
- Do care plans contain excessive abbreviations/meaningless subjective statements?
- Are regular ward meetings held to discuss the standards and progress of care delivery?

The questionnaire and audit data were analyzed, and the results helped to form a base for developing the teaching package used in the project.

Factors Inhibiting Implementation

The main inhibitor for the initiators of the project was felt to be a lack of knowledge about and understanding of nursing models. Sue Whittam, the key initiator, admitted that she and her nurse educator colleagues had to accept some of the blame for superficial teaching about specific models, which may have resulted in the rather skeptical views of the clinicians and managers. The diverse range of views and knowledge among staff, which the questionnaire and audit had uncovered, was revealing for Whittam and her colleagues.

Another point uncovered was that separation of the component concepts of the Roper-Logan-Tierney model (for example, some of the
nurses singled out only the Activities of Living and ignored the other
components) was useless if patients were to be considered holisti-
cally. Other potential inhibitors were resistance to change, evident
among some staff, and resentment at the inference that some further education about models might be helpful.

Factors Enhancing Implementation

Three main factors, according to Whittam, enhanced the implementation of the Roper-Logan-Tierney model. First, its implementation
was aided by the participation of some nurses who were already familiar with all components of the model and with the linkages
among its components. Second, there was a positive value in the enthusiasm of motivated, questioning, and innovative clinicians, educators, and managers. Third, the model was meaningful for nurses
whose central concern was for the patient/client.

Recommendations for Potential Implementers

In broad terms, five prerequisites are identified:

1. Securing an adequate level of interest across all spheres of the
   health care organization concerned, including nurse managers
   and lay administrators.
2. Involving managers in the development and ongoing progress
   (although some are relieved when nurse educators lead such
   initiatives, others may begrudge the educators' ability); they
   are the group who are currently most instrumental in supporting efforts to bridge the theory-practice gap.
3. Having initiators who are "knowledgeable salespersons" and
   can communicate clearly the benefits and purposes of integrating theory and practice.
4. Selecting the initial environment carefully and preparing key personnel to maximize the "cascading of expertise" through the organization (in the Manchester project,

education about the project eventually shifted from the college to in-service).

5. Sustaining the momentum: the more successful the progress, the more apparent the benefits become. Success breeds success.

Cost of Implementation

Although it was not done at the outset of this projeᶜt, the initiators now strongly recommend costing the proposed implementation of the model, including, for example, the costs of teachers' time, consultancy time (supportive and facilitative), starting and transfer, and monitoring the outcomes of implementation.

Goal Congruence/Conflict and Implementation

In terms of our model, the goals of nursing are: to consider the individuality of the patient/client in relation to the Activities of Living, irrespective of age and degree of dependence/independence in ALs, and to take into account the person's knowledge, attitudes, and behavior related to the ALs, as influenced by biological, psychological, sociocultural, environmental, and politicoeconomic factors. The function of nursing is to prevent, alleviate, solve, or help the patient/client to cope with problems (actual and potential) related to the ALs.

The project initiators consider that goal congruence exists when nurses utilize this conceptual framework (and, through it, also develop new knowledge) to the benefit of patients/clients. Goal conflict exists, they believe, when nurses are torn between the goals of client benefit and the goals of the organization, where cost efficiency displaces patient/client care as the crucial consideration.

SPECIFIC OBJECTIVES TO BE ACHIEVED IN IMPLEMENTATION

The specific goal of this project was to test the "theory" of the Roper–Logan–Tierney model in practice and to assess its effectiveness in relation to:

- Increasing nursing knowledge.
- Improving nursing practice.
- Providing theory to underpin practice.

Short-term results indicate that these objectives are being achieved, but the project is ongoing and the longer-term outcomes are yet to be assessed.

Time Line for Implementation

Initially, the project was developed by the key initiator over a 9–12-month period as a piece of academic work, but the total length of the project ran to 18 months. Monitoring and evaluation of the achievements are continuing via formal and informal processes.

Implementation: Assignment of Tasks

There were two main strands—educational and managerial. For educational purposes, college staff used formal clinical-education links throughout the hospital to publicize the project, prepare staff, and implement the project. In addition, the continuing education department within the service setting mounted series of courses related to new statutory regulations (UKCC) dealing with the importance of maintaining effective nursing records.

Nurse managers facilitated access to wards and departments, and to qualified nursing and nonnursing staff. Importantly, managers also negotiated access to the resources required. Without this input, the project could not have proceeded.

KEYS TO SUCCESS

A number of requisites for successful implementation of the model have already been mentioned. Sound knowledge and understanding of the model being implemented are absolutely essential, first on the part of the initiators and then among the users themselves. Enthusiasm and motivation to develop nursing practice, and in particular to strengthen its theoretical base, are also obviously essential.

The initiators are required to have leadership skills and to be willing to consult with, and listen to, the nurse managers and practicing nurses at every stage. In this project, the initial inquiry activities (i.e., the questionnaire and audit) probably set the correct tone, and collaborative links were maintained, as they must be, among practice, education, and management throughout the implementation phase and thereafter.

EVALUATION

Attempting a rigorous evaluation of the outcome of the implementation of a nursing model is a complex matter, even if this task were to be tackled by experienced researchers. Whittam has suggested that the outcomes of projects such as hers can be ascertained from a variety of sources, including:

- Nursing documentation.
- Nursing standards.
- Clinical audit.
- Educational audit.
- Patient satisfaction surveys.
- Staff appraisal.

Realistically, evaluation of the implementation of a nursing model is most likely to be a matter of informal, ongoing assessment by the implementers and the users of the model. It is fair to say that, if use of the model was *not* providing any benefits, the users would not persist with its implementation for long! The fact that the Manchester project has continued suggests that its implementers and its users believe that positive benefits have accrued from the introduction of the Roper-Logan-Tierney model.

REFERENCES

Audit Commission. (1992). *Making time for patients: A handbook for ward sisters.* London: HMSO.

Department of Health. (1993). *A vision for the future; the nursing, midwifery and health visiting contribution to care.* London: NHS Management Executive.

Fawcett, J. (1978). The 'what' of theory development. In *Theory development: What, why, now?* New York: National League for Nursing.

Fawcett, J. (1984). *Analysis and evaluation of conceptual models of nursing.* Philadelphia: Davis.

Flaskarud, K., & Halloran, E. (1980). Areas of agreement in nursing theory development. *Advances in Nursing Science, 3*(1), 1-7.

Jamieson, E. M., McCall, J. M., & Blythe, R. (1992). *Guidelines for clinical nursing practices related to a nursing model.* Edinburgh, Scotland: Churchill Livingstone.

Jourard, S. (1972). *The transparent self.* Reinhold: Van Nostrand.

Marriner-Tomey, A. (1989). *Nursing theorists and their work.* St. Louis: C. V. Mosby.

Meleis, A. (1985). *Theoretical nursing: Development and progress.* Philadelphia: J. B. Lippincott.

Reilly, D. (1975). Why a conceptual framework? *Nursing Outlook, 23,* 566-569.

Roper, N., Logan, W., & Tierney, A. (1980). *The elements of nursing.* Edinburgh, Scotland: Churchill Livingstone.

Roper, N., Logan, W., & Tierney, A. (1981). *Learning to use the process of nursing.* Edinburgh, Scotland: Churchill Livingstone.

Roper, N., Logan, W., & Tierney, A. (1983). *Using a model for nursing.* Edinburgh, Scotland: Churchill Livingstone.

United Kingdom Central Council for Nursing, Midwifery and Health Visiting. (1993). *Standards for records and record keeping.* London: United Kingdom Central Council for Nursing, Midwifery and Health Visiting.

Section VII

The Future

13

Theory Development: A Blueprint for the 21st Century

Afaf I. Meleis

A discipline's progress is measured by its theoretical developments and by the ability of its members to raise significant questions, to solve central problems, and to answer questions that have social significance. As a discipline, nursing is concerned with a unique set of phenomena, and it provides a specific perspective by which these phenomena are considered, examined, and developed. For a number of decades, nurse theorists have attempted to capture these phenomena and to develop frameworks to describe them. These theories of nursing have provided nurses with many opportunities to frame its problematics, systematically ask questions related to its phenomena, and uncover new phenomena that are germane to nursing.

The development of nursing theories during the past three decades has profoundly influenced the discipline of nursing in a number of areas. First and foremost, theoretical frameworks were used to strengthen nursing curriculum. Although the focus on the utilization of theoretical frameworks as structures for curricula and for course content may have been premature, and may have constrained the further development of substantive theory and nursing science, the process of considering the theories and operationalizing them may have contributed greatly to the development of theoretical approaches to teaching nursing.

Having these extant theories, and opportunities to consider and debate their utility, also influenced graduate education. In many nursing programs, theory may still be confined to theory and/or research classes; nevertheless, its presence in the program has allowed the students to experience theoretical thinking, practice theory application, and experiment with developing concepts. The extant theories in nursing affirmed to nurses that practice could be considered more abstractly and that some aspects of nursing have the potential of being considered theoretically. The theorists have also demonstrated, by developing their conceptualizations of nursing, the potential for nurses to think theoretically about nursing practice. When some nurses questioned the potential of any one theory in describing the whole of nursing, they began also considering whether all nursing practice could be captured in theoretical terms. The depth and complexity of nursing care stories demonstrated limitations of nursing theories in reflecting the whole of nursing care. Therefore, many thinkers in nursing made other contributions through concept analysis and development, and theory analysis and development. Concepts that have been proposed by nurse theorists as the cornerstones in their theories have transcended theories and have become central to the discipline as a whole. Examples are holism, self-care, caring, stress, external and internal environments, and responses, among others. This is demonstrated in *Nursing's Social Policy Statement* (ANA, 1995).

The mission goals contained in this social policy statement, which nurses have come to accept and use as a framework, were, I believe, driven, influenced, and made possible by the availability of nursing theories that have depicted the whole of nursing. The language and the concepts contained in the taxonomy of responses and actions could be traced to nursing theories, and I believe that, in analyzing it, we may be able to identify the thinking and the influence of nurse theorists on its development.

These first-generation theorists provided a number of frameworks for assessment and for identification of critical variables in the caring process. Their theories, however, were perceived to provide fewer guidelines for actions related to interventions. Finally, these theories have been instrumental in identifying and defining the concepts that are accepted as central in the discipline of nursing, such as environment, person, health, and nursing care.

There is very extensive literature demonstrating the utility of many of these theories in nursing practice. Some of this literature reflects individual nurses' use; other sources describe organizational use. Even when a single theory was not selected for use, there are many indications that the extant theories have stimulated many thoughtful theoretical discussions of nursing practice. These discussions have invariably resulted in value clarifications about theories, explorations of assumptions related to nursing care, and dialogues about the role of theory in practice, and vice versa. The process of participating in such discussions, a by-product of extant theories, may have contributed to clinical scholarship and collaboration between academics and clinicians.

THEORY FOR THE FUTURE

The task of developing theoretical frameworks that reflect clinical practice, better inform practice, and drive the research in the discipline, is not complete yet, nor will it ever be finished in dynamic and responsive disciplines (Meleis, 1992a). However, the goal for the development of theories and the means by which theories are developed may be refined and reconceptualized. The issues of the previous decade—defining the parameters of our domain, answering questions related to the essence of nursing, and/or articulating the discipline's mission—have been, to a great extent, resolved. This resolution is manifested through some cogent definitions of nursing and, most importantly, in the social policy statement (ANA,

1996). To continue to support the development of the discipline, the goals for the next decade must better fit the clinicians' vision for clinical practice, answer pressing societal questions about nursing care, and respond to the needs related to daily experiences of nurses and clients with health and illness.

Therefore, moving past definition of the discipline, a goal of the previous decade, we should be creating the means to refine health care and ensure that the knowledge developed will make a difference in clients' care. Two goals may bring the discipline closer to achieving this mission. The first goal is the development of situation-specific and context-relevant theories—theories that provide descriptions, explanations, and potential for prediction of and prescription for particular phenomena in more delimited situations. These theories would benefit from grand theories and from theories that are closer to practice than midrange theories are. The second goal is to endorse the development of the necessary appreciation and skills in thinking theoretically, by supporting the capabilities to do so and providing the means that allow members of the discipline to participate in theory development (Meleis, 1992b). There is great likelihood that the next wave of theories will be developed by a wider range of theorists, representing clinical practice, diverse populations, and a multitude of needs.

Given here are reflections on what the members of the discipline may want to consider to augment theory development, and some options for where the discipline's efforts on theory development may be directed. These proposals are intended to stimulate thinking, debate, and dialogue.

Integrative Theories

Nurses, the public, and the educators of the future will have become knowledgeable about the imperativeness and uniqueness of what nurses offer. With the increasing interdependence among disciplines, the need for knowledge that is relevant to a multiplicity of disciplines, and the decreasing boundaries between the roles of different health care professionals, we are faced with the challenge to revise existing theories and to develop new theories that reflect the integrative goals of health, wellness, and healing of our clients.

These integrative theories should be utilized by members of the health care teams who tend now to interchangeably play each other's roles—case managers, advanced nursing clinicians, and nurse practitioners, among others. Each of these roles depends on different bodies of knowledge. Some require different theories, such as theories for pain origins and pain management, or integration theories for symptom management. The primacy of knowledge for health care in general will become more imperative than the primacy of developing knowledge for a particular discipline. The challenge for nursing theory for the future is in the development of theories *for* and *in* health care. A number of health care professionals deal with similar phenomena in health care, such as pain, ulcers, presence, skin lesions, transitions, risk behaviors, styles of life, and many others. Each discipline may have a different perspective and each may have different priorities. However, together, the members of the different health care disciplines share some common goals: providing quality care, enhancing health, preventing disease, promoting wellness in illness, managing illness, and enhancing self-care. Each discipline, separately, is not capable of achieving these goals, nor should it be. However, common goals may require a common knowledge base and common theories. The challenge is to develop the strategies and processes that could support the development of common theories. Several current nursing theories could be considered as the bases for the development of more integrated theories. That integration will help put the patient together as a whole again and will allow the synergic nature of individuals and their environments to be manifested (Meleis, 1992c).

Several factors will drive the development of integrative theories. First, I believe that the uniqueness of nursing knowledge was an issue of the 20th century and was driven by the question generated during the 1950s: What is nursing? Theories evolved from attempting to answer this question. Second, drastic change is occurring in the health care system. Services and goals are changing as well, requiring patients to seek and accept care from health care professionals who have new roles (nurse practitioners, community workers, and family physicians). Third, there is an increasing recognition of the role of clinicians in the development of nursing knowledge. Collaboration between clinicians and academicians will allow a more careful consideration of the congruence of theoretical and clinical practice, and development of more clinically relevant conceptual knowledge. As a result, theories will be reconsidered, revised, and developed to reflect the germane questions and issues that clinicians experience in their daily work. Fourth, roles in the health care system are becoming interchangeable, and goals for health care are consolidating.

Theories that develop in partnership with other health care professionals (Bradshaw, 1995) and that evolve from existing theories and from a critical assessment of their tenets will mark the beginning of the next century. The blueprint example in this book illustrates conceptual compatability and integration.

Modification of Theories

The discipline of nursing is endowed with theories that were developed to address needs of patients, processes of nurse–patient relationships, the synergy between patients and their environments, and theories on health as an outcome. A number of well-developed classification systems are used for nursing diagnosis and nursing interventions. The future challenge for members of the discipline is to use these theories and classifications as a springboard for further development of theory. Each of these classifications and theories could be modified and further developed through exploration, clarification, analysis, integration, or reconceptualization. Some theory testing has been done, but theoreticians, clinicians, and academicians have been reluctant to propose revisions and modifications of existing theories. Several myths may have contributed to the limited theoretical revisions and to modification by other than the originators of the theories. One myth may be that the original theorists are the only ones who could modify or revise their theories, or that theories and/or classification systems could be modified, revised, or developed only after getting permission from the original theorists. Reluctance to request such permission could be a constraint. Some theorists may have perpetuated these myths by refusing to acknowledge modifications or by revising their theories themselves in response to critiques, rather than encouraging others, or their disciples, to undertake the modifications. Another myth may have been that theory modifications, revisions, and further development may only occur after the empirical testing and not through clinical narrative data or conceptual analyses of the theory. Our challenge is to facilitate the further development of existing conceptualizations and classification systems by removing obstacles and eliminating myths.

Theories and Informatics

We are moving steadfastly into an era when there will be client-centered information systems, organized data sets, and increasing availability of health care information to the public through network systems. Many aspects of people's lives will be dominated by computers. Our challenge is to address ways by which theoretical frameworks and informatics will interface. Hayes, Norris, Martin, and Androwich (1994) outlined the problems of adopting pluralistic philosophies in defining, connecting, and utilizing data and information for the purpose of practice, research, and policy development. There is equal concern about selecting one theory or classification system prematurely to guide these processes, but the risks may be higher in not settling on one shared framework. The challenge is to resolve these conflicts and to settle on a framework or frameworks that will facilitate exchanges and drive a more common and congruent set of outcomes. The challenge to face in the future is in the development of processes to integrate the development of informatic and theoretical nursing and to inform informatics with the mission, goals, and theories that reflect the discipline and the goals of health care. This challenge is beginning to be addressed, as is demonstrated in Chapter 11 of this book.

Development of Prescriptive Theories

Extant nursing theories, such as Neuman's, Johnson's, and Orem's, among others, provide a framework and guidelines to assess needs, problems, assets, and goals for nursing care plans. The prescriptive aspects of theories—that is, the guidelines for nursing actions and interventions—will become a challenging priority in the future. Clinicians may consider the utility of theories that reflect their daily practice in terms of the guidelines they provide for nursing thera-peutics. Such theories could provide guidelines for appropriate actions by caregivers. Prescriptive theories have several compo-nents—including a view of clients as whole, the integration of per-son–environment interactions, a consideration for energy levels, determination of levels of wellness, and person assets, among other components—that reflect theoretical frameworks. Prescriptive the-ories will provide options for interventions and will allow nurses' clinical judgment to determine the best course of action and the types of outcomes to consider.

Theories for Cultural Competence

With the increasing diversity of caregivers and clients, the increas-ing desire to maintain and disclose unique identities, and the height-ened awareness and demand of clients to receive quality care, there is urgent need for the development of culturally competent theo-ries. The urgency of this need is particularly generated by the heterogeneity of the U.S. population, which includes citizens repre-senting different countries of origin, ethnic backgrounds, religious preferences, sexual orientations, and gender identities. Further de-velopment of existing theories requires careful consideration and attention to the lived experiences of diverse populations and to op-tions for intervention that reflect diverse value systems, goals, and consequences. Similarly, testing of existing theories utilizing di-verse populations will support the further development of theories that are more culturally sensitive, and could provide options for ac-tion that may be more congruent with the heterogeneous needs of populations that are diverse. Moreover, theories addressing diver-sity may also address oppressions and ways by which to change and transcend present realities and rid clients of oppression in their en-vironments (Wuest, 1994).

Theories for Transitions

Health care delivery will continue to undergo some major changes, such as early discharges from hospital, more need for acute care at home, long-term care, urgency of continuity of care, and increasing need of care of the elderly at home or in institutions designed to emulate the home, and more need for rural care (Clarke & Cody, 1994; Long & Weinert, 1989). The care for these populations is characterized by the presence of more natural settings, community-based resources that are different from hospital resources, involvement of other personnel in the care, and changes in definitions and meanings of self-care, among others. More significantly, these changes will require the involvement of nurses in the care of families during the transition from hospital to long-term institutions, from hospital to home care, or from long-term institutions to other institutions. Nurses' roles will include facilitation of transitions for clients and their families. Each of the theories discussed in this volume could further be developed to encompass conditions and variables that best reflect the nursing care needs of these clients within the constraints of their changing environments as well as with utilization of the assets of their more natural surrounding environments.

Home care by nurses is becoming the wave of the future. Therefore, theories need to reflect the complexity of home and community in providing nursing care for clients. In the past, nurses have provided pioneering and innovative home care. Clinicians have consistently been concerned that the theories reflect more individual-focused care and less community care, and more focus on hospital settings and less on home- or community-based care. Future theories will be developed to provide guidelines for practice and research that incorporate conditions, variables, and goals that reflect the processes of transitions in health care and patterns of caring at home.

Theories for Global Nursing Care

There is empowerment in the unity of nurses internationally. Unity is enhanced by sharing a common mission and common goals, and by exchanging information. Developing and agreeing on goals, and being able to participate in information exchanges are predicated on having common symbols, if not common language. The symbols for nursing and in nursing cannot be generated by one group of nurses and transmitted to other nurses for utilization (Meleis, 1992c). It is more meaningful and powerful to have these symbols emerge from the collaborative efforts of nurses who represent different countries and reflect the diversity of clients' experiences and needs and the range of caring activities of nurses.

Nurses have attempted in many countries to utilize U.S.-generated nursing theories. Most of this utilization has been primarily in academic centers, less as frameworks for research projects, and even less in clinical settings. The major barrier to such utilization is the limited relevance of these theories to the daily lived experiences of nurses and to the experiences of patients in these countries. Instead of utilizing existing theories that reflect the U.S. value systems and contexts, there is a need to develop more internationally relevant theories as frameworks for testing, modifying, revising, and developing existing theories. The processes of theorizing and the theories developed by U.S. nurses during the middle decades of the 20th century have inspired similar processes in other countries. Many international colleagues have developed theories that are more relevant to their own countries; however, because of limited processes of dissemination, the utilization of these theories in the United States has been constrained. The reverse is not true. One international theory is discussed in this volume, marking the beginning of increased exchanges and reciprocity across cultures.

As nurses collaborate more internationally, and as reciprocation in knowledge development increases through computers and information exchanges, future development of theories will be more sensitive to varied client experiences and to the daily lives and actions of caregivers. However, to achieve this global perspective, there is a need for classification and maybe reconsideration of some fundamental assumptions that scholars hold. Clarification of assumptions and values occurs through collaborative work. Scholars need to assess the extent to which their belief in U.S.-produced theories has made them more valued than those developed by colleagues in their own countries.

Risks and Costs as Context for Theories

Diminishing resources in the health care system, and emphasis by health insurance agencies and health care administrators on financial costs of care, have necessitated the utilization of economic models and theories to drive health care assessment, actions, and outcomes. It is imperative to consider cost as both a significant variable and an outcome, in theories developed or utilized to guide processes of nursing. Future theorists are challenged to develop and refine theories with a consideration of the risks and costs inherent in the use of a particular theory, as well as its benefits.

Most of the current theories lack guidelines for assessment and determination of financial costs and/or rewards for using the theories, beyond those that are expressed in terms of health. Financial costs and rewards have rarely been considered in developing conceptualizations about nursing. Whether cost and reward variables could be developed as components of theories, or whether they should be considered in the utilization of a theory for research and/or practice, is a question that begs careful analysis. It is clear, however, that future knowledge development must incorporate and demonstrate more attention to risks and costs, particularly when budgets and financing have preceded the expenditures. Chapter 2 begins to adddress this with new approaches to use of the Neuman Systems Model.

CONCLUSION

We are entering a new era for knowledge development and for testing and advancing knowledge (Shaw, 1993). It is an era in which scholars are accepting that clinicians have an important role to play in developing knowledge, clinicians are more trusting of the knowledge that scholars are describing and generating, and nurses in general are tending to trust their own intuition, observations, and judgments. It is also an era in which theories will be legitimized for use, not only because they were empirically tested, but because they receive support through philosophical and conceptual analysis, anecdotal description of their utility, and stories that demonstrate the meanings attributed to practice from theory and vice versa (Meleis, 1995).

Nursing as a discipline, and nurses as clinicians, educators, and researchers, will continue to need theoretical and conceptual thinking. The need for seeing situations as wholes and attempting to bring order to a world that is complex and chaotic will never cease to be a goal in all disciplines. Unified conceptualizations of nursing practice, a characteristic of nursing theories, will always occupy nurse scholars; however, whether such conceptualization will be developed by nurses and will depict nursing phenomena through nursing theories or through interdisciplinary theories remains as a challenge of the future.

In the meantime, we must empower clinicians, researchers, and new-age theorists by opening up extant theories for modifications, alterations, and further development (Caroselli, 1995). As Reed (1995) advanced, by ensuring that there are no closed ideologic systems, we will ensure that the "dialogue on knowledge development continues into the 21st century" (p. 82).

The theories that were developed by nurses during the decades of 1950–1980 have helped in transforming nursing to its paradigmatic status. As we approach the 21st century, we are assured that the domain of nursing is focused on the whole of individuals, their experiences, and their relationship with their environments; and on nurses and their interactions in bringing about a sense of well-being for patients. We approach the next century with conceptualizations and knowledge that empower nurses to make a difference in patients' lives. The more conscious nurses are of the theories they use in their practice, the more they are aware of their options for theories, and the more they recognize their own role in expanding, clarifying, and developing theories, "the more readily they will be able to enter into a transformative relationship with clients" (Newman, 1994, p. 156; Newman, Lamb, & Michaels, 1991).

This volume celebrates the continuing progress in the development, utilization, and testing of nursing theories. The challenge for future theorists is to continue with the mission of theory development.

REFERENCES

American Nurses Association. (1995). *Nursing's Social Policy Statement.* Washington, DC: American Nurses Publishing.

Bradshaw, A. (1995). What are nurses doing to patients? A review of theories of nursing past and present. *Journal of Clinical Nursing, 4,* 81–92.

Caroselli, C. (1995). Power and feminism: A nursing science perspective. *Nursing Science Quarterly, 8*(3), 15-119.

Clarke, P. N., & Cody, W. K. (1994). Nursing theory-based practice in the home and the community: The crux of professional nursing education. *Advances in Nursing Science, 17*(2), 41-53.

Hayes, B. J., Norris, J., Martin, K. S., & Androwich, I. (1994). Informatics issues for nursing's future. *Advances in Nursing Science, 16*(4), 71-81.

Long, K. A., & Weinert, C. (1989). Rural nursing: Developing the theory base. *Scholarly Inquiry for Nursing Practice: An International Journal, 3*(2), 113-132.

Meleis, A. I. (1992a). Theoretical thinking progress in the discipline of nursing. In K. Krause & P. Astedt-Kurki (Eds.), *International perspectives on nursing.* Tampere: University of Tampere Department of Nursing, pp. 1-12.

Meleis, A. I. (1992b). Nursing: A caring science with a distinct domain. *Sairaanhoitaja,* 8-12.

Meleis, A. I. (1992c). Directions for nursing theory development in the 21st century. *Nursing Science Quarterly, 5*(3), 112-117.

Meleis, A. I. (1995). Theory testing and theory support: Principles, challenges, and a sojourn into the future. In Betty Neuman (Ed.), *The Neuman Systems Model* (3rd ed., pp. 447-457). Norwalk, CT: Appleton & Lange.

Newman, M. A. (1994). Theory for nursing practice. *Nursing Science Quarterly, 7*(4), 153-157.

Newman, M. A., Lamb, G. S., & Michaels, C. (1991). Nurse care management: The coming together of theory and practice. *Nursing and Health Care, 12,* 404-408.

Reed, P. G. (1995). A treatise on nursing knowledge development for the 21st century: Beyond postmodernism. *Advances in Nursing Science, 17*(3), 70-84.

Shaw, M. C. (1993). The discipline of nursing: Historical roots, current perspectives, future directions. *Journal of Advanced Nursing, 18,* 1651-1656.

Index

Achievement (subsystem, JBS Model), 34
Activities of living (ALs), 293-297
    model for nursing, 289. *See also*
        Roper-Logan-Tierney Model
Adaptation:
    concept of Levine's Conservation Model,
        191-192
    modes of (four), 69
Adaptation level theory (and Roy Adaptation
        Model), 66
Administration, use of nursing models in:
    Neuman Systems Model, 251-274. *See also*
        Neuman Systems Model (NSM)
        psychiatric facility, 262-273. *See also*
            Psychiatric facility, implementation of
            Neuman Systems Model
        public health agency, 253-262. *See also*
            Public health agency, implementation
            of Neuman Systems Model
    Riehl Interaction Model, 241. *See also* Riehl
        Interaction Model
    Self-Care Deficit Nursing Theory
        (computerization of), 275-286. *See also*
        Self-Care Deficit Nursing Theory (S-CDNT)
Affectional adequacy, 71
Affiliative (subsystem, JBS Model), 34
Aggressive/protective dependence (subsystem,
    JBS Model), 34
AIDS Lobby for Better Living, 168
Allentown, PA, Lehigh Valley Hospital, 221
Allentown College of St. Francis de Sales, 219, 222
ALs, *see* Activities of living (ALs)
Alverno Health Care Facility, 218, 220
Annual Rocky Mountain Regional Conference
    on HIV Disease, 168
Areas I-VI, *see* Blueprint(s)
Associate degree, and Neuman Systems Model,
    91-140. *See also* Neuman Systems Model
    (NSM)
    assessment, 119
    assumptions, 107-108
    client populations, 110-112
    concepts/subconcepts of model, 101, 103-104
    diagram (Neuman Systems Model), 98

diagram (student as center of system), 111
enhancement and inhibitions to
    implementation, 121-122
evaluation, 131-132
fit, determining, 109
implementation, 94, 115
philosophical relationship of model to
    setting/user, 96, 97
planning, 121-122
preparation of faculty, students, and staff, 113
resources needed, 118
structure of model, 105
Australia, 144, 181

Baccalaureate degree, and Neuman Systems
    Model, 91-140. *See also* Neuman Systems
    Model (NSM)
    assessment, 118-119
    assumptions, 107
    client populations, 110
    concepts/subconcepts of model, 99-101, 103
    enhancement and inhibitions to
        implementation, 119-121
    evaluation, 130
    fit, determining, 108-109
    implementation, 92-94, 114-115
    philosophical claims of Neumann College
        Nursing Program Faculty, and major
        concepts (Appendix A), 138-140
    philosophical relationship of model to
        setting/user, 95-97
    planning, 119-121
    preparation of faculty, students, and staff,
        112-113
    resources needed, 116-118
    structure of model, 104-105
Baycrest Center for Geriatric Care, 167,
    169-172, 180
BBARNS (Boston Based Adaptation Research in
    Nursing Society), 84
BCFs (basic conditioning factors; Self-Care
    Deficit Nursing Theory), 276
Behavioral system model, *see* Johnson
    Behavioral System (JBS) Model

Birmingham, Alabama, 42
Birthing center pilot study (primary
    prevention/secondary prevention), 27
Blueprint(s):
    for administration, *see* Administration, use of
        nursing models in
    determining fit of particular model, 1–10
    for education, *see* Education, use of nursing
        models in
    example of using (integrated model for
        evaluation, research, and policy analysis
        in context of managed care), 11–30
    international, 289–314. *See also*
        Roper-Logan-Tierney Model
    outline form, 4, 5–9, 17, 21, 26, 28
    overview description, 1–10
    for practice, *see* Practice, use of nursing
        models in
    references, 9–10
    for research, *see* Research, use of nursing
        models in
Boston Based Adaptation Research in Nursing
    Society (BBARNS), 84
Brazil, 144, 181

California, University of, Survey Research
    Center, 43, 45
California State University, 91, 132–133
Canada, 144, 251
    Baycrest Center for Geriatric Care, 167,
        169–172, 180
    Collaborative Nursing Education Project, 180
    Doctors' Hospital, 167
    Elizabeth Breyere Health Center, 274
    hospitals in, using caring theory as
        foundation for clinical nursing, 167
    Ontario, College of Nurses of, 254
    Princess Margaret Hospital, 167
    Saskatchewan, University of, 133
    Standards of Nursing Practice for Community
        Health Nurses in Ontario, 254, 257
    Toronto, University of, 171
Caring Assessment Tool, 176
Caring Behaviors Inventory (CBI), 177
Caring competencies/modalities/strategies, 173
Caring documentation instrument (CDI), 178
Caring theory, *see* Transpersonal Caring,
    Watson's Theory of
Catholic University Nursing Faculty, 230, 276
CBI (Caring Behaviors Inventory), 177
CDI (caring documentation instrument), 178
Cecil Community College, Maryland, 92, 94. *See
    also* Associate degree, and Neuman
    Systems Model
Chicago, *see* Illinois, University of, at Chicago,
    College of Nursing
Children, chronically ill:
    research project, studying activities of,
        33–63. *See also* Johnson Behavioral
        System (JBS) Model
    variables influencing activities of, 34–41
Children's Hospital, Denver, 174
China, Republic of, 144
Chronic illness:
    in children, and research project, *see*
        Children, chronically ill

in women, *see* Levine's Conservation Model,
    use in practice—care of women with
    chronic illness
CNC, *see* Rochester, University of, School of
    Nursing, Community Nursing Center (CNC)
Cognator subsystem (and coping mechanisms),
    68, 78, 79
Collaborative Nursing Education Project,
    Victoria, 180
Colorado:
    Center for Human Caring, 179–181
    Children's Hospital, Denver, 174
    Denver General Hospital, 168
    Denver Nursing Project in Human Caring,
        167–169
    Denver Veterans Hospital, 168
    University Hospital, Denver, 168
    University of, School of Nursing, 164,
        167–169, 172
Community Nursing Center, (CNC), *see*
    Rochester, University of, School of Nursing,
    Community Nursing Center (CNC)
"Comprehensive" *vs.* "holistic" (NAP survey), 27
Computerization of Self-Care Deficit Nursing
    Theory, 275–286. *See also* Self-Care Deficit
    Nursing Theory (S-CDNT)
Conservation model, *see* Levine's Conservation
    Model
Contextual stimuli (and Roy Adaptation Model),
    67–68, 77, 79
Coping Checklist, Revised Ways of, 78
Coping mechanisms (and Roy Adaptation
    Model), 68

Darby, PA, Mercy Catholic Medical Center, 274
Del Webb Hospital, 174
Denver General Hospital, 168
Denver Nursing Project in Human Caring,
    167–169
Denver Veterans Hospital, 168
Department of Health and Human Services
    (DHHS), 168
Dependence/independence continuum, 299–300
Doctorate, nursing (N.D.), 163
DSCRs (developmental self-care requisites; Self-
    Care Deficit Nursing Theory), 276

Edinburgh, University of, 292
Education, use of nursing models in:
    Neuman Systems Model, 91–140. *See also*
        Neuman Systems Model (NSM)
    Riehl Interaction Model, 241. *See also* Riehl
        Interaction Model
    Watson's Theory of Transpersonal Caring,
        141–184. *See also* Transpersonal Caring,
        Watson's Theory of
Eliminative (subsystem, JBS Model), 34
Elizabeth Breyere Health Center, 274
England, 144, 181, 290. *See also* Manchester
    project
Englewood Hospital, 174
Environment:
    and Conservation Model (commonplace of),
        194–195, 207–208
    metaparadigm (person/environment/health/
        nursing), 92, 304

and Neuman Systems Model, definitions, 102
and Roy Adaptation Model, 67-68
Evaluation:
    and blueprint, 5, 9, 28
    Levine's Conservation Model (practice), 217
    Neuman Systems Model (administration),
        260-261, 271-272
    Neuman Systems Model (education), 130-132
    Riehl Interaction Model (practice), 246-247
    Rogan-Logan-Tierney Model (international),
        313
Excellence in Government Awards Program,
    169

Family (variable influencing children's
    activities), 37-39
FANCAP mnemonic, 240
FCDs (foundational capabilities and
    dispositions; Self-Care Deficit Nursing
    Theory), 276
Fibromyalgia (FM), 192, 204-214
Fit, determining (of model), 1-10
Fitzgerald Mercy Division, 274
Florida, Holmes Regional Medical Center, 174
FM, see Fibromyalgia (FM)
Focal stimulus (and Roy Adaptation Model),
    67-68, 77, 79
FONE Functional Independence Measure, 78
Future, blueprint/recommendations for, 12,
    317-329. See also Theoretical
    developments, nursing

General systems theory (and Roy Adaptation
    Model), 66
Gil's Model for Social Policy Analysis (GMSPA),
    17, 19-21, 22-26
    integration with Neuman Systems Model
        (chart), 13
GMSPA, see Gil's Model for Social Policy
    Analysis (GMSPA)

Hartford, CT, Mt. Sinai Hospital, 274
Hawaii, Kuakini Health Care System, Honolulu,
    274
HDSCRs (health deviation self-care requisites;
    Self-Care Deficit Nursing Theory), 276
Health:
    commonplace of Conservation Model, 195
    metaparadigm (person/environment/health/
        nursing), 92, 304
Helene Fuld Health Trust, 164
HIV/AIDS, 168
Holism (and Roy Adaptation Model), 66
"Holistic" vs. "comprehensive" (NAP survey),
    27, 28
Holmes Regional Medical Center, 174
Humanism (and Roy Adaptation Model), 66
Humber College, 171

Iceland, St. Joseph Hospital, 274
Illinois, University of, at Chicago, College of
    Nursing, 221
    Rockford Program, 172-173
Indiana State Board of Health, 230
Indiana University-Purdue University, 131
Indonesia, 144

Ingestive (subsystem, JBS Model), 34
Instruments available for research:
    drawbacks, 81-82
    modification of, 82
Integrated model for evaluation, research, and
    policy analysis in context of managed care
    (blueprint example), 11-30
Interaction Model, see Riehl Interaction Model
Interdependence (mode of adaptation), 69, 71,
    79
International blueprint, see
    Roper-Logan-Tierney Model

Japan, 144, 181
JBS Model, see Johnson Behavioral System (JBS)
    Model
Jefferson Davis Memorial Hospital, 274
Johnson Behavioral System (JBS) Model, 33-63
    references, 59-63
    research project, chronically ill children, 33,
        41-59
    scholars working with, 59
    subsystems (six), 34
    summary, 52-55
    variables that influence children's activities,
        34-41

King's Daughter Hospital, 174
Korea, 144, 181
Kuakini Health Care System, 274
Kuwait, 144

Lehigh Valley Hospital, 221
Levine's Conservation Model, 187-227
    acknowledgments, 223
    assumptions, 202-203
    concepts/subconcepts:
        concepts, 191-194
        relationships among, 197-198
        subconcepts (commonplaces), 194-196
    conclusion, 220
    curriculum development—nurse scholars
        who can assist (names/addresses/phone
        numbers), 220-221
    description, brief, 188-189
    evaluating use of, 217
    examples of successful uses of, 204
    implementation, 217-220
    philosophical basis, 189-203
        purpose of model, 191
        theoretical background, 189-190
    practical aspects, 203-204
    references, 223-227
    strategic planning, 214-216
    structure, 198-202
    success tips, 216-217
    use in practice—care of women with chronic
        illness, 204-214
    values, 203
Living, activities of, see Activities of living (ALs)
Living, model of (diagram), 294
LJNMEI (Lowry-Jopp Neuman Model Evaluation
    Instrument), 131
Logan, see Roper-Logan-Tierney Model
Lowry-Jopp Neuman Model Evaluation
    Instrument (LJNMEI), 131

McMaster University, 171
Managed care context (blueprint example),
  11–30
Manchester project, 290, 305–306. *See also*
  Roper-Logan-Tierney Model
Medical Clinics of Houston, 174
Medicus Patient Classification Tool, 176
Mercy Catholic Medical Center, 274
Metaparadigm (person/environment/health/
  nursing), 92, 304
Middlesex-London Public Health Nursing
  Division, 253–262. *See also* Public health
  agency, implementation of Neuman
  Systems Model
Minnesota, 133, 292
Models:
  applications of:
    Gil's Model for Social Policy Analysis
      (GMSPA), 17, 19–21, 22–26
    Johnson Behavioral System (JBS) Model,
      33–63
    Levine's Conservation Model, 187–227
    Neuman Systems Model (NSM), 17–19,
      21–22
    Riehl Interaction Model, 236–248
    Roper-Logan-Tierney Model, 289–314
    Roy Adaptation Model, 64–87
  and National League of Nursing, 131
  scope, broad (four tasks of), 113–114
Montreal, Université de, Faculté des Sciences
  Infirmières, 167
Montreal General Hospital, 167
Mt. Carmel Hospital, 174
Mt. Sinai Hospital, 274

NAP, *see* National Academy of Practice (NAP)
Natchez, MS, Jefferson Davis Memorial
  Hospital, 274
National Academy of Practice (NAP), 27
National Council Licensure Examination
  (NCLEX), 119
National League of Nursing, and models, 131
NCLEX (National Council Licensure
  Examination), 119
Neighborhood (variable influencing children's
  activities), 39–40
Neuman-Gil Model for Evaluation, Research,
  and Policy Analysis (development/
  implementation; blueprint example), 11–30
  chart of integration of models, 13
  background, 14–17
Neumann College, 91, 92–94
Neumann College Nursing Process Tool, 110
Neuman Notes, 260
Neuman Systems Model (NSM), 17–19, 21–22,
  91–140, 251–274
  applied to administration, 251–274
    psychiatric facility, 262–273. *See also*
      Psychiatric facility, implementation of
      Neuman Systems Model
    public health agency, 253–262. *See also*
      Public health agency, implementation
      of Neuman Systems Model
  applied to education, 91–140
    associate degree, *see* Associate degree, and
      Neuman Systems Model

baccalaureate degree, *see* Baccalaureate
  degree, and Neuman Systems Model
client populations, 110
evaluation, 130–132
fit, determining, 108
implementation, 92–94
philosophical claims of Neumann College
  Nursing Program Faculty, and major
  concepts (Appendix A), 138–140
resources needed, 116–118
success factors/tips/strategies, 128–130
support needed, 125–126
target audience, impact of, 123–125
assessment, 118–119
assumptions, underlying basic (ten), 105–107
concepts/subconcepts, 97–99, 101–104
diagram of model (original), 93
examples of use of, 132–133
expert assistance available, 115
implementation examples, 118–125
  philosophical relationship of model to
    setting/user, 95–108
  theoretical underpinnings, 95
purpose of model, 96
references, 133–137
scope/complexity of, 113–114
strategic planning, application of principles
  of, 126–128
structure, 104
terms objectionable, NAP Survey, 27
Neuman Systems Trustees Group, Inc., 115, 116
Nevada, University of, 133
Newark Beth Israel Medical Center, 228, 229,
  230, 275–286
New Jersey Department of Health, 280
  Nursing Incentive Reimbursement Program,
    230, 280, 281
New Zealand, 144, 180
NIS, *see* Nursing information system (NIS)
North Dakota, 133
NSI, *see* Nursing Systems International (NSI)
NSM, *see* Neuman Systems Model (NSM)
"Nurse" *vs.* "provider" (NAP survey), 27
Nursing:
  and application of models:
    administration, *see* Administration, use of
      nursing models in
    education, *see* Education, use of nursing
      models in
    practice, *see* Practice, use of nursing
      models in
    research, *see* Research, use of nursing
      models in
  commonplace of Conservation Model, 195–196
  metaparadigm (person/environment/health/
    nursing), 92, 304
  model for (diagram), 295
  profession/discipline, 146
  theoretical developments in, *see* Theoretical
    developments, nursing
Nursing Audit Tool, 261
Nursing Development Conference Group, 230,
  276
Nursing information system (NIS), 276. *See
  also* Self-Care Deficit Nursing Theory
  (S-CDNT), computerization of

Nursing Systems International (NSI), 233, 276, 281
Nurturance (sustenal imperative), 35, 58

Oklahoma State Department of Health, 274
Ontario, College of Nurses of, 254
Orem's Self-Care Deficit Nursing Theory, see Self-Care Deficit Nursing Theory (S-CDNT)
Ottawa, Ontario, Canada, Elizabeth Breyere Health Center, 274

PAIS-SR, see Psychosocial Adjustment to Illness Survey, Self-Report (PAIS-SR)
Patient Satisfaction Visual Analog Scale, 176
PCs (power components; Self-Care Deficit Nursing Theory), 276
Peers (variable influencing children's activities), 39
Person:
    commonplace of Conservation Model, 194
    metaparadigm (person/environment/health/ nursing), 92, 304
Physiologic adaptation, and Roy Adaptation Model (table), 79
Physiological (variable influencing children's activities), 36-37
Physiologic needs (mode of adaptation), 69-70
Portugal, 144, 181
Practice, use of nursing models in:
    Levine's Conservation Model, 187-227. See also Levine's Conservation Model
    Riehl Interaction Model, 236-248. See also Riehl Interaction Model
    Roper-Logan-Tierney Model, 289-314. See also Roper-Logan-Tierney Model
    Self-Care Deficit Nursing Theory (S-CDNT), 228-235. See also Self-Care Deficit Nursing Theory (S-CDNT)
Princess Margaret Hospital, 167
Protection (sustenal imperative), 35
"Provider" vs. "nurse" (NAP survey), 27
Psychiatric facility, implementation of Neuman Systems Model, 262-273
    critical path to model implementation, 264-273
    facility—Whitby Mental Health Center (WMHC), 262-263
    historical considerations, 263-264
    staff responses, 263-264
    references, 273
    resources/contacts, 274
Psychosocial Adjustment to Illness Survey, Self-Report (PAIS-SR), 79
Public health agency, implementation of Neuman Systems Model, 253-262
    evaluation, 260-261
    goals, 257
    language of model, 255
    Middlesex-London Public Health Nursing Division, 253-254
    planning, 255-256
    records, nursing, 261
    references, 273
    resources/contacts, 274
    selection of model, 254
    success, key factors for, 259-260
    summary, 261-262
    support, 256-257
    time line, 258-259
Purdue University, 131

Redundancy, Theory of, 200, 201
Regulatory subsystem (and coping mechanisms), 68, 78, 79
Rehabilitation Hospital of Montreal, 164
Rehabilitation nursing, research study, and Roy Adaptation Model, 64-87. See also Roy Adaptation Model
Research, use of nursing models in:
    integrated model (Neuman-Gil), for evaluation, research, and policy analysis, in context of managed care, 11-30
    Johnson Behavioral System (JBS) Model, 33-63. See also Johnson Behavioral System (JBS) Model
    Riehl Interaction Model, 241. See also Riehl Interaction Model
    Roy Adaptation Model, 64-87. See also Roy Adaptation Model
Residual stimulus (and Roy Adaptation Model), 67-68, 77, 79
Riehl Interaction Model, 236-248
    analysis of tasks/people, 245-246
    assessment of model in use, 242-243
    assessment of organizational setting, 243-244
    assumptions, 244
        analytic, 237-238
        genetic, 238-239
    complexity of, 242-247
    concepts/processes, 239-241
    evaluation of model in practice, 246-247
    experts, availability of, 242
        resource contacts (names/addresses), 248
    explanation of model, 236-239
    fitting conceptual model to practice setting, 241-242
    language, 244
    philosophical underpinnings, 236-239
    planning, 244-245
    references, 247-248
    success, ensuring, 246
    time/cost/training factors, 242
Rochester, University of, School of Nursing, Community Nursing Center (CNC), 14-17, 274
    challenges in selecting and implementing a nursing theoretical model, 14-15
    components for success, 15
Rockford Health System, University of Illinois at Chicago, College of Nursing Rockford Program, 172-173
Role function (mode of adaptation), 69, 70-71, 78
Roper-Logan-Tierney Model, 289-314
    applicability of model in practice setting, 304-305
    assumptions, 302-304
    components of, 293-302
    description of, 293-304
    evaluation, 313
    evolution of, 291-293
    general application, 305-307

Roper-Logan-Tierney Model *(Continued)*
  patient/client populations, intended, 306
  simplicity of model, 306-307
  implementation, 307-312
  introduction, 289-291
  metaparadigm concepts, relationship with,
    304
  references, 313-314
  success, keys to, 312-313
Roy Adaptation Model, 64-87
  applying, step-by-step approach to, 82-83
  as basis for research, 71-74
  overview, 66-71
  practical aspects of, and fit within nursing
    research and practice, 81-83
  references, 85-87
  rehabilitation nursing, research study,
    75-81
  research, use in, 83-85
  summary, 85
Rykov Hospital, Jonkoping, Sweden, 274

St. Joseph Hospital, Reykjavik, Iceland, 274
San Francisco, 42
Saskatchewan, University of, 133
SCA (self-care agency; Self-Care Deficit Nursing
    Theory), 276
Scandinavia, 144
S-CDNT, *see* Self-Care Deficit Nursing Theory
    (S-CDNT)
SCOLs (self-care operation limitation
    statements), 280
SCOs (self-care operations; Self-Care Deficit
    Nursing Theory), 276
Scotland, 144
Scottish Highlands Center for Human Caring,
    180
Self-Care Deficit Nursing Theory (S-CDNT),
    228-235, 275-286
  applied to administration, 275-286
  applied to nursing practice, 228-235
  assumptions, underlying, 231-232, 278, 282
  computerization of, 275-286
  concepts/subconcepts, 230, 276-277
  fit, 278
  implementation, 232
  phases (five major), 234
  proposition, basic, 230
  references, 235, 285-286
  structure, 231, 276
Self-concept (mode of adaptation), 69, 70, 78
Seneca College, 171
Sequelae of Spinal Cord Injury Instrument, 78
Sexual (subsystem, JBS Model), 34
Sickness Impact Profile, 176
Sigma Theta Tau International, 168
SMSA (Standard Metropolitan Statistical Area),
    42
Social policy analysis, *see* Integrated model for
    evaluation, research, and policy analysis in
    context of managed care (blueprint
    example)
Social Policy Statement, 318

Spinal cord injury, 68, 69, 74-75. *See also* Roy
    Adaptation Model, rehabilitation nursing,
    research study
Standards of Nursing Practice for Community
    Health Nurses in Ontario, 254, 257
Stimulation (sustenal imperative), 35, 58
Strong Memorial Hospital, 26
Survey, National Academies of Practice (NAP),
    27-28
Survey Research Center, University of
    California, 43, 45
Sustenal imperatives
    (protection/nurturance/stimulation), 35,
    55-56

Temple University, 221
Tennessee, University of, 133
Texas, University of, at Arlington, School of
    Nursing, 222
Theoretical developments, nursing:
  conclusion, 327-328
  future, 319-327
  past (general), 317-319
  references, 328-329
Therapeutic Intention, Theory of, 200-201
Tierney, *see* Roper-Logan-Tierney Model
Toronto, University of, 171
TQM (total quality management), 171
Transpersonal Caring, Watson's Theory of,
    141-184
  background, 143-145
  caring paradigm, 147-151
  cosmology/worldview for, 145-151
  examples of model in action, 162-181
  philosophical underpinnings, relation to
    practice, education, research, 145-147
  practical implications, 160-162
  references, 181-184
  theory content, 151-160
TSCD (therapeutic self-care demand; Self-Care
    Deficit Nursing Theory), 277

University Hospital, Denver, 168
USCRs (universal self-care requisites; Self-Care
    Deficit Nursing Theory), 276

Veritivity (and Roy Adaptation Model), 66
Victoria University Department of Graduate
    Nursing and Midwifery, Wellington, New
    Zealand, 180

Watson's theory of caring, *see* Transpersonal
    Caring, Watson's Theory of
Whitby Mental Health Center (WMHC),
    262-263. *See also* Psychiatric facility,
    implementation of Neuman Systems Model
Wholeness (concept of Levine's Conservation
    Model), 191, 193-194
Wholistic *vs.* holistic, 95
Winter Haven Hospital, 174
Women with chronic illness, caring for,
    187-227. *See also* Levine's Conservation
    Model